The Double Brain

The Double Brain

STUART DIMOND
M.A., B.Sc., Ph.D.

Lecturer in Psychology
University College, Cardiff

Churchill Livingstone
Edinburgh and London

1972

To Bridgit

First published, 1972
ISBN 0 443 00900 7

Printed in Great Britain by
The Whitefriars Press Ltd., London and Tonbridge

Preface

'One of the most obvious facts about the human cerebrum is that it is double. One hemisphere is structurally the gross mirror image of the other. That is, the other side is not only structurally the same, but is working just as hard. I submit that the informational capacity of one is just as great as the other, or put differently, the other side is not only working just as hard but also just as intricately' (Bogen, 1969a).

This view of function is one which has emerged recently as the result of modern studies of the brain which separate one hemisphere from the other by section of the cerebral commissures—the system of fibres interconnecting the cerebral hemispheres. Not all authors agree that one hemisphere is the equivalent of the other, even in respect of the amount of work carried out, and the views of Bogen may have to be qualified to some extent. Nevertheless, this book presents the evidence for a two-brain point of view and shows that it is useful to approach the problems of the nervous control of function through this concept. It discusses the hemispheric organizations which, through their own individual contribution and through their integrated activities, provide the underlying machinery for the control of both normal and pathological behaviour.

The two-brain system is investigated here in the light of much work which combines the approach of experimental psychology with that of clinical neurology and other neurosciences. The origins of this book lie in experiments carried out by the author which examine the two-brain system of man. These emphasize the importance of joint function and interaction in performance in relation to the behaviour of the normal person. They also point to similarities and differences between the functions of one hemisphere and the other.

Optic fibres from the temporal half of the retina pass to the hemisphere on the same side of the body. Fibres from the nasal retina cross the midline to join the opposite hemisphere (Guyton, 1966). Messages can be directed separately, some to one hemisphere and others to the opposite hemisphere. Alternatively messages can be directed two at a time to the same hemisphere, either the right or the left. The experiments used signals for reaction time—letters, numbers and words—and these were projected at the same time, one to each hemisphere, or both to the same hemisphere, either the right or the left. From these studies it became clear that similarities between the hemispheres are important, as are the differences, and that the picture of brain function which supposes that particular functions are exclusive to one hemisphere or that the brain is a unilateral mechanism is not supported by the facts.

These studies also suggest a flux and interplay between the hemispheres. The attribution of functions to the right or the left, stating that the right does this or the left does that, may be an oversimplification. Integration of activity becomes important when it is considered, as the studies show, that the brain as a whole is able to enhance its performance if some at least of the load is distributed. Integration may not come about immediately on receiving information. The evidence suggests that each hemisphere analyses separately the information presented to it before sharing with the other. In other words, there is in the brain a double perceptual analysing system and the use of two hemispheres may often be better than the use of one.

The picture of brain function which emerges is that of a two-brain individual in which each half-brain analyses separately the information it receives. The total capacity of the brain is different from that which might be assumed by supposing that the brain carries out only one function at a time, or that it consists only of a single channel of limited capacity. The study of normal human brain processes as a two-brained system is only just beginning. The experiments to date do not allow us to specify the nature of the system in any great detail, but at the same time they point to an arrangement in which there is both individuation as well as an interaction between one half of the system and the other.

From the earliest evolutionary developments of the nervous system along bilateral lines we witness the emergence of a duplicated structure, which in infra-human species also shows duplicate function. Evidence comes from studies of spreading cortical depression, hemispherectomy, unilateral lesion, and studies of commissure section. The two-brain system is prominent from the earliest origins of bilateral organisms. It is an impressive feature of the vertebrate nervous system. How far does the two-brain arrangement persist as a feature of the human nervous system? As regards physical appearance, the basic bilateral pattern has not changed. The question of how far this is also true of function is the one to which we address ourselves in the following chapters.

Stuart Dimond
June, 1972

Acknowledgements

In the preparation of this manuscript I was extremely fortunate in having the advice and criticism of Professor J. Z. Young, F.R.S. His paper *Why do we have two brains?* provided the initial stimulus for this work. It has been a privilege to draw on his critical faculties and extensive knowledge of the literature.

Professor O. L. Zangwill has been especially helpful in his criticism and encouragement. He has read the complete manuscript and the book has benefited from his insight and wisdom. His published papers, quoted as they are throughout the text, have been a constant source of inspiration.

Professor G. Westby also read the complete manuscript, and I am grateful not only for his criticism but for the opportunity of discussion and for his help in facilitating the research on which the manuscript is based.

I am greatly indebted to those eminent investigators who kindly agreed to read individual chapters—Professor R. W. Sperry who read the chapters on *Hemisphere Disconnection in Animals and Man* concerning the split-brain work developed under his brilliant guidance; Professor R. C. Oldfield who read the chapter on *Language*; Professor I. S. Russell who read the chapter on *Spreading Cortical Depression*; Dr. J. McFie who read the chapter on *Hemispherectomy*; and Professor Doreen Kimura who read the chapter on *Laterality*. Their knowledge, insight and criticism have proved most valuable to my work. No responsibility of course attaches to any of the former for the shortcomings of this book.

I am sincerely grateful to those friends and colleagues who have given so generously of their time and effort, and also to those who helped prepare the manuscript. Mrs. S. Hudson and Mrs. P. Jones were remarkably patient in transforming a difficult handwritten account into type. Finally, I thank my wife who has assisted at every stage of this book, and has remained calm and encouraging even during the most difficult phases of its preparation.

Contents

1

Evolution of the Double Brain

CEPHALIZATION

Some of the difficulties of controlling large networks of sensitive and conducting cells may be overcome by the natural progressive tendency of certain regions of the nervous structure to predominate over others. This is particularly apparent in the tendency of the head to occupy a dominant position over the more lateral parts of the nervous system. The head usually contains a dense concentration of sense organs, and it is not surprising, therefore, that it also encloses the associated centres of nervous control.

The principle of head dominance plays an increasingly important role with the concentration of the nervous elements and the enhanced complexity of the sensory systems. The forward local centre now takes a greater part and with the advent of rapidly conducting nervous tissue, this effective area of domination becomes considerably extended. It has been argued that one of the greatest advances in evolution was the acquisition of the simple habit of moving head first (Dethier and Stellar, 1961). Not only does this initiate a more complex feeding process, which is accompanied by the development of the necessary neuromuscular coordinates, but it also entails the distribution of most of the major sense organs within the anterior region. The major organs for exploration have moved into the positions of greatest prominence where they will be most effective. The accompanying nervous support systems become concentrated in the head region, and integration of function is facilitated by the emergence and amalgamation of these separate systems into what is later to become the brain.

Cephalization brings with it the grouping and rearrangement of the major nervous control systems into the principal ganglia of the head. Head dominance becomes a more and more important feature as the phyletic scale is ascended. Another remarkable feature, to which we shall return, is that the brain of animals occupying a cephalo-dominant position on the phyletic scale is double, usually composed of two major ganglia and several subsidiary ganglia lying on either side of the gut. In these animals the nervous system takes the form of a double nerve cord stretching back from the head region to the rest of the body, so that each half of the conjoint brain and nervous system forms the mirror image of the other.

1

It seems likely that the tendency towards cephalization, and the movement of the sense organs into an anterior position, were responsible for this development. The first organisms representative of this type lived in water, a medium in which the chemical senses are particularly important. The moving animal needs to sample the environment before entering it. There are two important factors here. First the organism, if it is to use the sense organs to their full advantage, needs to be able to detect the spatial position or the spatial direction of the chemical stimuli. Secondly the organism needs to be able to orientate its body movements in relation to the source of the stimuli. If, for example, we consider the search for food by a mobile organism living in a fluid medium, chemical stimulation from food reaching the anterior sense organs on one side of the head must evoke the responses which lead the animal to turn towards the source of food. The concentration of substance as gauged by the organ at one side may be greater than that sensed by the other. If the message is directed to the brain on the same side of the body, the brain can operate the muscles on that side, leading the organism to turn directly towards the food. In having two brains and two nervous systems, left and right, each acting on different messages received from sense organs, the animal is able to locate objects in space, e.g. food objects, and move rapidly towards them. The double brain can be seen as a primitive but important system for mapping the environment (Young, 1962). It is also a system which directs the movements of the organism towards a particular spatial localization.

THE PRIMITIVE DOUBLE NERVOUS SYSTEM

From an early point on the phyletic scale organisms are to be found which are, in all major respects, symmetrical about a central body axis. The nervous system too is notable for its bilateral symmetry, and for the fact that in structure it is double appearing as two separate strands running along each side of the body, interconnected only by lateral commissures.

The development of rapid nerve conduction permits an increase in body size, but there are still limits to the efficiency of nervous conduction. The double system, operating within a bilaterally symmetrical framework, ensures that no one part of the body is too distant from the source of effective nervous control.

It is unrealistic to think of the nervous system in isolation. The limited size of the organism imposes strict requirements for micro-miniaturization, and if some organs already occupy most of the available space, then others have to be accommodated around them. The gut, for example, holds a prominent central position. The nervous system can most conveniently straddle the gut, its major ganglia lying on either side. In this way the nervous system receives physical support, which it would not do if it occupied a central position at the top of the gut. Factors such as mechanical support and the necessity to occupy that space which is available cannot be overlooked when considering the development of the nervous system.

The suggestion that the double or tandem nature of the nervous system is fundamental in this and succeeding stages of evolution receives support from a study of representative phyla of the animal kingdom. In relatively primitive organisms, e.g. the freshwater mussel (*Anodonta*) and similar members of the family, the nervous system is composed of only a small number of ganglia and their interconnecting commissures. Nevertheless it is a paired structure.

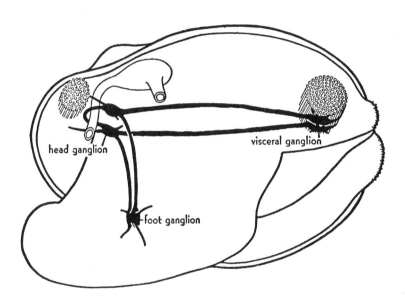

Fig. 1. The nervous system of the clam has a pair of ganglia for each main region of the body. The head ganglia correspond to the double but fused 'brain' of other animals. They lie on each side of the mouth, joined by a connective that runs around the oesophagus. They send nerves to palps, anterior shell muscle, and mantle. From each head ganglion, a connective runs ventrally to the ganglia which supply the muscles of the foot. Two connectives also run from the head ganglia to the visceral ganglia, which send nerves to the digestive tract, heart, gills, posterior shell muscle, and mantle. (From *Animals without Backbones* by Ralph Buchsbaum, 1938. Chicago: University of Chicago Press.)

There are three principal pairs of ganglia—the cerebral, located near the oesophagus; the pedal, located within the muscular foot; and the visceral near the posterior adductor muscle. These ganglia are sometimes described as though each was a single structure, but this is not the case. Inspection shows clearly that they are double and that the nervous system itself is paired.

In some of the most primitive worms (flatworms, Planarians) the pattern of nervous arrangement follows a symmetrical plan. These animals have two enlarged cephalic ganglia, forming protuberances at the anterior end. Longitudinal nerve strands lead back from the ganglia, which act as receiving and distributing systems. Both sides of the

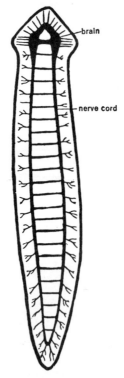

Fig. 2. Nervous system of a planaria. (From *Animals without Backbones* by Ralph Buchsbaum, 1938. Chicago: University of Chicago Press.)

nervous system are connected by commissural fibres. Here, in what is known as the 'ladder type' of nervous system, we have certain fundamental features which are capable of further development—a system of potential.

The 'ladder type' of nervous system shows marked bilateral symmetry. Furthermore, it is in anatomical terms an obvious double structure, each half the mirror image of the other. Structural features which may have contributed to this double form have already been discussed, and it may be that these alone were responsible for the basic morphology. However, even in such relatively primitive organisms as the flatworms, we can discern elaboration of nervous mechanisms which not only share the labour of control, but also provide additional support should common mechanisms fail, either through some intrinsic breakdown, or through accident or injury.

The annelids or segmented worms of the type similar to the common earthworm are much more highly organized than the flatworms. The nervous system for the most part is synaptic. Most nerve cells are concentrated in a double chain of ganglia located on the ventral body wall, one pair of ganglia to each segment of the body. The two ganglia of each segment are connected to one another by means of a fibrous commissural strand, and to the corresponding ganglia of the adjoining segments by longitudinal fibre connectives. The whole nervous system resembles a rope ladder, the ganglia forming an accumulation of nerve cells at the points where the rungs and struts cross.

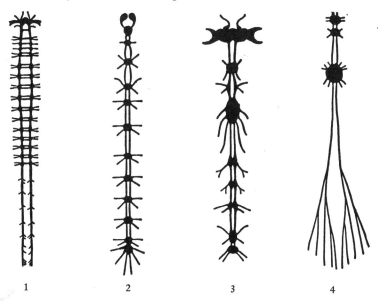

1   2   3   4

Fig. 3. Nervous systems of various arthropods, showing fusion of the ganglia. 1. Primitive crustacean. 2. Caterpillar. 3. Honeybee. 4. Water bug. (From *Animals without Backbones* by Ralph Buchsbaum, 1938. Chicago: University of Chicago Press.)

The bilaterally symmetrical ladder type of nervous system is found in the segmented worms, the crustaceans, the spiders and the insects. In some cases the pattern may be obscured because the ganglia occur in close proximity or in some cases may have fused, but usually the double structure is visible. Not all organisms conform to this double plan. Echinoderms show a very clear radial symmetry. So also do sessile worms, e.g. *Myxicola,* but here it is the exception which proves the rule since radial symmetry has to be abandoned in favour of bilateral symmetry when head first movement is used, in some forms, as the typical means of progression.

THE VERTEBRATE BRAIN

The embryological development of the vertebrate brain follows a surprisingly similar course throughout the classes. In advance of any development in the nervous structure, a body polarity is laid down and the nervous system shaped to accord with pre-existing gradients. The nervous system itself first appears as a thickened plate of ectodermal epithelium along the mid-dorsal surface of the body. This becomes folded inwards to form a trough, and then, as the processes meet, a tube which becomes separated from the outer skin. The neural folds gradually approach each other until they meet and fuse in the midline. The neural tube develops and separates itself from the outer skin. There is usually some enlargement in the region of the head, which is a typical expression of its relative importance.

The epithelial tube of the trunk becomes the spinal cord; the cephalic portion undergoes more radical change and develops protuberances to become the brain. In essence both the spinal cord and the brain retain something of their tubular quality throughout life, the interior containing the cerebro-spinal fluid, essential to the regulation of the surrounding nervous tissue.

Originally the nervous system takes the form of a hollow cylinder. Its later diversity is reached by growth of the various outfoldings of the walls of the tube. The cerebral hemispheres are themselves an outgrowth. They represent the most extravagant unfolding of the system. The neural tube develops from the upward growth of two bilaterally symmetrical neural folds, which develop by a folding and thickening of the tissue in their walls. The fact that a hollow area exists and persists through the mid-region serves to emphasize rather than disguise the division between one side of the brain and the other.

The simultaneous advancement of the central vertebrate skeletal structure has not been without effect on the nervous system it contains. The skeletal structure precludes the possession of a double spinal cord.

However, while that part of the nervous system posterior to the brain shows a great deal of unification in vertebrates, physical differentiation between one side of the spinal cord and the other is still a principal feature. It is even possible that each half of the spinal cord retains autonomy over its separate functions. Although we may acknowledge then that skeletal influences have exerted a unifying effect, the brain generally appears to have resisted this tendency. Throughout the vertebrate phyla the cerebral regions maintain their paired structure, and the morphological division by which each separate half acts as the partner of the other is characteristic.

EVOLUTION OF THE FOREBRAIN

Amongst the chordate group it is possible to trace the development of the nervous system from primitive to sophisticated forms. In *Amphioxus,* a small fish-like creature, the nerve cord (which is little more than a primitive tube) runs forward to the head. There is no substantial evidence of specialization here and the brain as such does not really exist. The development of skeletal material around the central nerve cord appears to have suppressed the typical bilateral nervous structures.

The nervous system of *Amphioxus* shows no sign of the functional subdivisions which are to feature at a later date. Sergeev (1964), for example, showed that the animal reacts equally to various stimuli, whether they occur at the head or tail, and when the nervous system was divided surgically into several segments, temporary conditioned response connections could be established in any part of the nerve tube, both anterior, posterior and centrally.

Among higher vertebrates, differentiation of the various divisions of the central nervous system is more marked. In the lamprey, however, some diffuse modes of response are still preserved. For instance, when the forebrain and optic lobes are excised, conditioned reactions to light and other stimuli remain. But these conditioned responses tend to be relatively unstable (Baru, 1955).

The development of the brain as a paired structure becomes more obvious in other fish. We see the development of the powerful paired suprasegmental apparatus of the cerebellum. Swimming and active procurement of food bring a need for refined spatial discrimination as well as advanced control over motor functions. The existence of two large areas of brain—the double structures of the cerebellum—plays a considerable part in this and surgical removal of the cerebellum can impair learning performance.

Fundamental changes take place in brain organization following migration from an aquatic to a terrestrial form of life. The

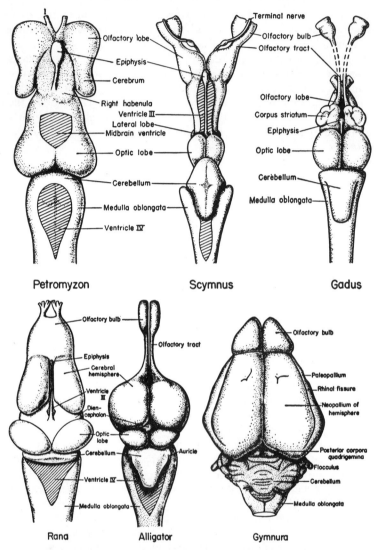

Fig. 4. *Upper,* dorsal views of the brain of a lamprey, a shark, and a teleost (codfish). Hatched areas are those in which a choroid plexus has been removed, exposing the underlying ventricle. *Lower,* dorsal views of the brain of a frog, an alligator, and a tree shrew. (From *The Vertebrate Body* by A. S. Romer, 1962. Philadelphia and London: W. B. Saunders and Co.)

distance-receptor system is elaborated and certain changes in the brain relative to its double structure may be associated with this. In the amphibians, however, the major development has yet to occur. As far as can be judged, the amphibians occupy a stage in which the cerebellar integration system undergoes regressive changes, while at the same time other newly formed mechanisms are in a rudimentary state. Sergeev (1964) presents evidence that the overall level of brain function is reduced and that regressive changes also occur in the cerebellum.

Below the reptiles in the evolutionary scale, there is no cerebral cortex. Diamond and Hall (1969) point out that the modern reptiles show some concentration of neurones on the surface of the cerebral hemispheres, but this represents only a primitive state of development and there is still doubt as to whether the neocortex, a feature of the development of mammals, exists in even a primitive form in the reptiles (Filimonoff, 1964).

The evolution of the paired structures of the neocortex is the feature which largely distinguishes the brain of mammals from other vertebrates. Some of the earliest mammals show surprisingly advanced cerebral development when the neopallium is considered. The cerebral hemispheres are relatively large, and it is possible that in such animals as the duck-billed platypus (*Ornithorhynchus*) and the spiny anteater or echidna (*Tachyglossus aculeatus*), the development of the brain has reached an advanced state. On the other hand, it may be that in the development of the major paired system of the cerebral hemispheres, there are other factors which must be taken into account besides the function of the neopallium as an association area. For example, the prefrontal region of the cerebral cortex may be concerned with the ability to maintain body temperature independent of surroundings (Fielding, 1968).

It is commonly supposed that the laying down of later tissue during the course of development of the vertebrate brain is a means of enhancing the powers of analysis and integration. It is suggested that the sensory systems and their cerebral machinery are adequate at first for the task of carrying out appropriate discriminations, but additional tissue allows refinement over and above this in terms of the power to resolve events and to compute and anticipate for the future.

Towards the front end of the cerebral cortex, a new evolutionary step has occurred. In primitive mammals there is a major expansion of the neopallium which spreads out to cover the top half of the cerebral cortex and provides for more sophisticated brain function. The underlying brain structure has crystallized. The development of the neopallium provides a means of expanding brain size as well as capacity,

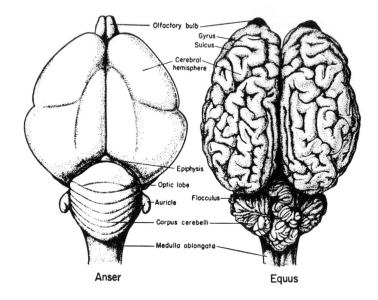

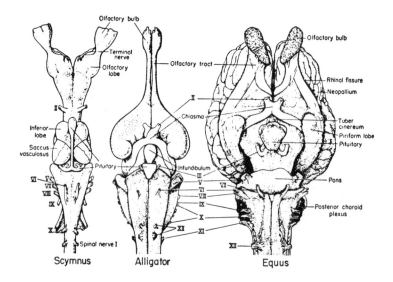

Fig. 5. *Upper,* dorsal views of the brain of a goose and a horse. *Lower,* ventral views of the brain of a shark, an alligator, and a horse. (From *The Vertebrate Body* by A. S. Romer, 1962. Philadelphia and London: W. B. Saunders and Co.)

without disturbing the more primitive organizations lying beneath. From this complex superstructural apparatus arise new modes of nervous activity.

Diamond (1967) argues that the neocortex is the most conspicuous and characteristic feature of the mammalian brain. It would appear to be the area responsible for the behavioural processes which distinguish higher mammals from other species. He also argues that the crucial step in the origin of the neocortex is the penetration of sensory fibres from the diencephalon into the hitherto olfactory-dominated pallium. The mammalian series shows an enormous increase in the ratio of non-olfactory to olfactory cortex. In an ascending series of living primates—tree shrew, lemur, monkey, apes and man—the regions intercalated between the primary sensory cortex, the so-called association cortex, expand while the sensory areas of the thalamus and cortex appear stable. This is a dramatic development in primates, which overshadows other features.

However, we must not ignore the size which the mammalian brain ultimately attains. In some animals the growth of the neopallium outstrips development in other brain regions. Thus in evolutionary terms this area becomes one of the most active centres of change. Some of the large animals have correspondingly large brains—the brain of a whale, for example, may be four times that of a man—but much brain space appears to be devoted to the direct control of muscular and other somatic functions, so that little remains for other purposes. However, if the brain is large relative to the body, then this forms one major advance in the production of intelligent behaviour.

A sharp rise in brain mass is to be observed in the higher primates, and indeed many of the smaller monkeys show a larger mass for their size than do human beings. Even so, in modern man the brain at birth is almost as large as that of a full-grown orang-utan. In maturity the average weight of the human brain is 1,450 grams, giving a brain-body ratio of 1 : 50. This development takes place mainly in the massive double cerebral hemispheres with their large areas of association cortex.

Some of the characteristic features of the human brain may be a direct consequence of its increase in size and weight. The paired organs of the cortex are more deeply and extensively fissured than that of most lower forms. This could be explained by the fact that, whilst the total volume of the cortex increases roughly as the cube of the weight of the brain, the average thickness of the cerebral cortex of primates remains fairly constant (von Bonin, 1950; Bok, 1959). With large brains this may be a developmental necessity.

It is important to emphasize other factors besides those of size and weight. In many cases the relationships of mass have been emphasized at the expense of the significance of restructuring or organization.

Holloway (1968) quotes the clinical condition of microcephaly as illustration of this. People with remarkably small brains display the typical features of human behaviour and appear not to be as seriously handicapped as might otherwise be supposed. Throughout the vertebrate division the major cerebral regions of the brain maintain their paired structure, and the morphological division into two separate halves is a remarkable feature of its structure.

PROBLEM OF CROSSED LATERAL CONTROL

In considering the basic paired design of the invertebrate system, it seems reasonable to suggest that the nervous structures on one side of the body exert a large measure of control over the motor functions of that same side. The double brain may be viewed first as a system for spatial analysis, but more importantly in this context as one for steering and guiding bodily movement. The invertebrate system is not only a double system but to a large extent a local one.

If the vertebrate system followed the same plan, typified by the 'ladder nervous system', we might expect each hemisphere also to control its own lateral half. Yet the evidence is overwhelming that the domain of hemispheric control in the vertebrate system is not the lateral half of the same side but that of the opposite side. There are many ways in which the vertebrate brain differs from the invertebrate brain, but one of the most remarkable is the fact that it has crossed lateral control of movement. Fritsch and Hitzig (1870) showed, for example, that electrical stimulation of points along the precentral gyrus on one side of a dog's brain gave rise to movements on the contralateral side. This finding has been confirmed by a number of subsequent investigations (Ferrier, 1876; Liddell, 1955).

Crossed lateral control creates a problem when we consider how the vertebrate nervous system arose from more primitive forms. What is its significance in the organizational history of the brain? It seems to point to the possibility, speculative as this may be, that there has been a functional interchange of control between one hemisphere and the other. It would be going beyond the evidence to suggest that this was the result of structural rotation, nevertheless it remains a possible explanation of the particular functional arrangement.

In the early ladder system, it is not difficult to see that a functional interchange of ganglia could occur by rotation of the brain through 180° relative to the rest of the nervous system. This would preserve the connections of each half of the brain to each half of the body. If each limb is a fixed reference point, and the invasion of embryonic nerve tissue towards it is equally unchanging, it seems that the reorganization took place in the brain and not in systems linking the brain to the rest of the body.

The arrangement of the sensory systems also suggests something of this. The sensory apparatus of mammals consists of crossed projection fibres—powerful systems for transmission of information from the sense organs to the cerebral hemispheres. The ipsilateral fibres, where they have developed, tend to be weaker and less efficient. Milner (1962) suggests not only that the auditory projection fibres from the ear to the opposite hemisphere are more fully developed in most mammals, but also that they function in a more effective manner. The crossed visual fibres are also more fully developed. As far as is known the fibres of the optic nerves of all primitive mammals cross over or decussate completely at the optic chiasma (Walls, 1963). In these organisms, each eye projects its information completely to the opposite side of the brain. In animals somewhat more advanced ipsilateral fibres are present, but those linking the eye to the opposite hemisphere are more effective than the ipsilateral fibres (Nadel, 1966). In advanced mammals with frontal eyes and an overlapping binocular field, part of the retina on the temporal side sends fibres to the optic tract on the same side and therefore to the ipsilateral hemisphere.

When the eyes occupy a forward position, as in cats and human beings, effective connections come to be sent to both hemispheres of the brain. It is possible nonetheless to show that the nerve cells of the visual cortex are more sensitive to messages from the opposite eye than from the eye on the same side. Blakemore and Pettigrew (1970) argue that stereoscopic vision may depend on the difference between the two projections. However, to show a difference of response is not the same thing as showing that this is essential to stereoscopic vision. It could as well be that the difference indicates that the mechanisms controlling depth perception are still to some extent underdeveloped, and that the full potential of the visual system for binocular vision has not yet been achieved.

Be that as it may, this finding illustrates the superiority of the crossed lateral fibres and suggests that they are primary, both in the sense of being most efficient, and in the sense of being the first to be laid down. This evidence again suggests an interchange of function, and taking the sense organs as fixed reference points, indicates a reorganization or rotation of brain structure, as well as secondary development of the projection fibres.

It is difficult at first sight to see what advantage this functional interchange confers. The crossover points might be expected to coordinate input and output from the two hemispheres, but in fact do not appear to do so. Most coordination is achieved through cross-talk between one hemisphere and the other by way of the corpus callosum.

An alternative view, which seems more likely, concerns the relationship of the nervous system to the external world. Throughout evolution the sensory systems have become more sophisticated. Primitive eye spots appear to be concerned with diffuse light detection, but even these may be used for spatial localization, and light detectors situated at strategic points upon the body can give a clear indication of the direction of illumination. Even simple visual systems may have potential for elementary spatial analysis. Events occurring to the left of the organism stimulate the receptors on that side, so that correspondence exists between the source of stimulation, the receptor stimulated and the movement made in response to the stimulus.

It has been argued previously that the double brain arose in response to the demands for a system which allows the organism both to differentiate factors in space and to orientate bodily movement towards particular spatial positions (Young, 1962). The functions of a sensory system could be enhanced if, instead of indicating only the direction of a stimulus source, it were possible to pinpoint the distance of the source from the organism and thus define its exact locus in space. The perception of distance is a refinement of sensory organization, and the presence of paired sense organs with comparison of the input to each seems to be the means by which this is achieved.

Young (1962) has argued that one important reason why we have two brains is connected with this role of binocular vision. It should be pointed out, though, that a double nervous system is a feature of many primitive organisms which have not yet evolved binocular vision. So whilst it seems reasonable to suppose that the appearance of binocular vision played some part in the development of crossed lateral control, the existence of the double brain cannot be attributed entirely to this source.

Sokolov (1960) has argued that the organism constructs a neuronal model which mirrors, in neural terms, the spatial arrangement of the world about it. In other words it acts as an analogue of the external world. In the primitive state, spatial correspondence is maintained in the chain of nervous control between the stimuli and the responses which relate to them. Young (1962) has pointed out that the advanced vertebrate eye inverts the retinal image. It also shows another feature, and that is that it reorders space. Events appearing to the left are registered to the right of the eye and vice versa. If representations of the spatial world ,are to correspond with brain locus, and perhaps equally important, with the functions of the lateral motor systems, then reorganization may be essential to compensate for transformations introduced by the eyes. Even amongst the most primitive vertebrates possessing eyes of the typical vertebrate pattern, we find crossed lateral visual projection.

Lampreys are somewhat unusual in that they pass through a larval state in which the photoreceptors are not paired. These animals show non-directional response to visual stimulation. The presence of light causes them to bury themselves in the mud. Whereas the adult has fully developed paired eyes and crossed lateral projection, the optic nerves from the eyes cross completely ending in the central and lateral quadrants of the tectrum (Stöer 1940). Young (1962) argues on the basis of this and other evidence that paired receptors and paired brain structures are necessary to preserve the isomorphic relationship between the events of the world and their registration within the brain.

It seems likely that the double brain arose in association with bilateral body symmetry and that the lateralization of motor control played a significant part in the development of the system as it now is. The question of the origin of crossed lateral relationships is a different one from that of the origin of the nervous system as a double structure. Whilst crossed lateral control can be regarded as a reorganization of brain structure engendered by the development of sensory systems which confer advantages on the organism possessing them, the double brain itself appeared prior to this and, in terms of the origins, appears to relate even more significantly to the organization of bilateral motor control.

SIGNIFICANCE OF THE CORPUS CALLOSUM

Throughout the evolution of the brain there has been a tendency for advancement to occur by the progressive laying down of fresh tissue on pre-existing structures. This has meant that changes have been most frequent in the anterior dorsal regions. Deposition of fresh tissue on pre-existing structures carries the implication that some areas have a greater potential for change than others. The more primitive structures exist in a relatively stable form, having been laid down at an early point in time, whereas more recent structures may not yet have established their final pattern.

The cerebral cortex occupies one of the topmost positions on the brain and is of recent development. Assuming that spatial restrictions apply to the total volume which the brain may occupy, and assuming that the thickness of the cerebral cortex is limited by its requirements for nutrition and respiratory gas interchange, it could well be that the cortex has already achieved its full potential. There is room, however, for advancement within the existing double system of the cerebral hemispheres and this would not impose the same demands as thickening of the cortical tissue or expansion of the brain cavity. This

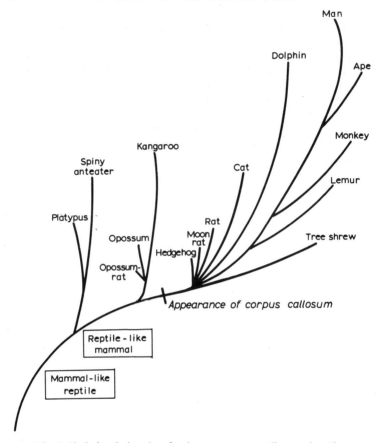

Fig. 6. Phyletic relations in a few important mammalian species. The height of the various lines of descent attempts to suggest the expansion of neocortex relative to old cortex. (Diamond, 1967. In *Contributions to Sensory Physiology*, edited by W. D. Neff. New York: Academic Press.)

advancement lies in the sophistication of the fibres which link the cerebral hemispheres—that is the interconnecting commissures which bring about integration by coordinating the activities of one half of the brain with the other.

Major developments have ensued from wedges of tissue interposed between more imposing structures. Filiminoff (1964) points to the corpus callosum in this respect, as an interleaving tissue between the hemispheres. It may represent not only a recapitulatory and primitive system, but also an important growth point from which further developments have taken place. What is more, this area has come to play an important part during the recent history of the brain.

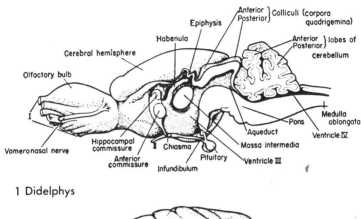

1 Didelphys

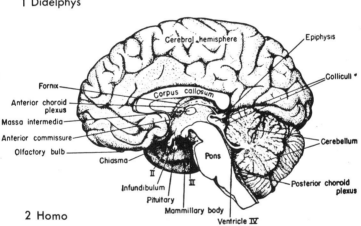

2 Homo

Fig. 7. Right half of the brain (median aspect) of: 1. An opossum (after Loo). 2. Man. Unshaded areas are those sectioned. The internally bulging side walls of the diencephalon may meet and fuse in the midline, forming a 'mass intermedia' which, however, has no functional importance. (From *The Vertebrate Body* by A. S. Romer, 1962. Philadelphia and London: W. B. Saunders and Co.)

The marsupial brain, whilst truly mammalian in structure, is of a simple and generalized type compared ,with higher forms. It is of interest because of the rudimentary nature of the corpus callosum, if it exists as such at all. It has been shown that the anterior commissure in these animals fulfils the function of lateral brain integration (Putnam *et al.*, 1968), and provides also for trans-hemispheric integration.

The development of the corpus callosum, and other commissural systems, strengthens the capacity for cross-talk within the brain. During evolution a major increase in the size and functional importance of the corpus callosum is observed, although at the same time it must be remembered that in some of the lower primates there are still fairly large areas of neocortex which have anterior commissure connections rather than callosal ones. Whitteridge (1965) suggests that the efficiency of the callosal connections relates to the fact that the visual field is split through the area of most distinct vision in the more advanced organisms, and that the development of the corpus callosum is a product of retinal specialization for forward vision. The horse and other ungulates have eyes in which the region of splitting does not involve the area of most distinct vision; therefore callosal connections are less well developed. In the cat and the monkey callosal connections assume more complex forms, and these animals have a split in the visual field through the fovea. Transmission times reach their fastest rate in the callosum of man (Whitteridge, 1965) and it is possible to trace the increasing importance of the corpus callosum in terms of the speed with which information is passed across it.

Although it can be argued that this development is related to the need for integration of visual function, it is clear that the callosum also transports other types of information, and may be regarded as an essential general transport system across the brain.

There are differences between species in the physical structure of the corpus callosum, in the speed of conduction, and in the density of inter-hemispheric connections. Using the technique of strychnine neuronography, the connections from one side can be traced to the homologous area in the opposite hemisphere, as they pass through the interconnecting commissural regions. The patterns of fibre degeneration, following total section of the corpus callosum and the anterior commissure, can be demonstrated. The racoon has relatively few cross-connecting fibres compared with other animals. There are no commissural fibres relating to the distal zones of both fore and hind limb extremities, and there is also a complete absence of fibres relating to the sensory area of the forepaw (Welker and Seidenstein, 1959). There is an absence of commissural projection for the visual cortex and those parts of the body which are most used for exploratory and anticipatory functions also fail to receive commissural projections. Some parts only of the auditory cortex have projections, but even these bear no relationship to known patterns of function. Somewhat similar considerations apply in the case of the cat, although clearly the density of cross-connecting fibres is very much greater than in the racoon.

In the monkey far more widespread degeneration occurs in the cortex after total commissure section. The occipital lobe degeneration closely resembles that seen after contralateral occipital lobectomy. The commissural systems in the monkey contain densely packed fibres which, with a few exceptions such as the auditory receptive area and the hand and foot region of the parietal lobe, interconnect all major areas of the cortex on one side with those of the other. In tracing development upwards through the phyletic scale, we see elaboration of the corpus callosum as a structure which increases in importance and one which acts through the density of its fibres to bring about more and more efficient coordination between the two major regions of the brain. In man this interconnecting system is very large indeed and represents a major advance in efficiency. By increasing the capacity for cross-talk within the brain, elaboration of function is made possible without any major increase in the space which the brain must occupy.

Is evolutionary development still taking place in this area? This depends on whether the brain as a whole is continuing to evolve. If it is, then it would be expected that developments beyond those already achieved would take place in the corpus callosum.

CONCLUSIONS

We have seen in this chapter how the nervous system as we know it made an early appearance as a double system, with duplicate nerve chains and duplicate ganglia, but soon developed into the typical 'ladder' pattern we find represented in the Planarians. This basic plan has remained unchanged throughout the invertebrate phyla.

Among the major vertebrate groups we also see a brain which is double, and not only double but deeply divided in its structure. The question arises, then, why did it evolve in this way? What are the factors which prevented its coalescence at an early stage?

Young (1962) argues that the brain has to map the events of the outside world, and that a double brain is better than a single brain at preserving these isomorphic relationships. He suggests that another factor is the retinal image which is inverted by the lens of the vertebrate eye. A double brain allows the retinal image to be reinverted and thus preserves spatial equality. In addition it should be pointed out that the double nervous system is a feature of organisms which existed long before the vertebrate eye evolved. Crossed lateral control therefore might have the function of reinverting the retinal image, but this alone cannot explain why the organism effectively has two brains. Double representation and crossed lateral projection of information is a feature of the auditory nervous system, and here there is no lens acting to invert the auditory image.

It might be argued that the double nervous system is essential for the proper perception of space and distance. By matching the input from different sense organs, the organism is able both to determine the direction of a stimulus source and to calculate its distance. But does this necessarily demand a functional separation of brain areas? Probably the answer is yes, if confusion between different spatial images is to be avoided, since the double system in separating images helps to preserve their integrity.

Perhaps a more fundamental reason for a double brain stems from the fact that most living organisms have a double body, that is, they show bilateral symmetry. If one side of the body is to be activated independently of the other, for example limb function, then it is essential that systems of control are evolved which are to a large extent spatially separate, so that messages to one limb will not be confused with those to the other. Feedback information about body function and limb movement must reach the brain too. It would be pointless to deal with this centrally since it relates specifically to a particular limb on one side of the body only.

While stressing the important phylogenetic development of the double system, it must not be forgotten that connections do exist between the two halves of the brain and that in vertebrates there has been a progressive advance in its size and complexity as well as in the speed of function of the commissural fibres which link the two cerebral hemispheres.

2

Spreading Cortical Depression

INTRODUCTION

The concept of duplicate function within the brain can be investigated by studying the effects of spreading cortical depression. As a technique it allows us to examine the functional value of the cortex. By alternate depression of each hemisphere in turn, the degree to which the functions of one resemble the functions of the other may be fully assessed. The nature of neocortical transfer of information is determined by training one hemisphere in isolation, and then testing the other after reversal of the depression. This method can also be used to study the way in which the two hemispheres integrate their function. Much of the work described in this chapter lends support to the view that the brain exists as a duplicate system of control. It discusses the problem of whether each hemisphere is invested with sufficient effective machinery to control behaviour on its own account. In fact, is each hemisphere largely capable of independent function? Does each half form the functional mirror image of the other, and is this shown, as far as animals are concerned, in most major functions which the hemispheres are called upon to perform?

DESCRIPTION OF THE EFFECT

The technique of spreading cortical depression provides a powerful tool for investigating the relationship in performance of one hemisphere to the other. It owes its inception to the work of Leaõ (1944) who showed that cortical function may be depressed for a period of time by the slow spread of a wave of electrical activity. This may be induced by strong repetitive electrical stimulation applied at a particular point on the cortex. The wave of electrical activity expands from its point of origin to increasingly distant parts of the cortex. This is shown by simultaneous recording from several pairs of electrodes. The wave which travels at the rate of 2—3 mm per minute, temporarily suspends the activity of all the neurones in its path. It is accompanied by a negative after discharge which reaches a magnitude of approximately 10 millivolts at its peak (Leaõ, 1947).

21

The rate of recovery is relatively slow. After the wave has spread, it takes several minutes (sometimes more than ten) before the spontaneous electrical activity of a particular cortical area returns to normal in all of its regions.

Electrical stimulation is not the only means by which to elicit spreading cortical depression. It may also occur in response to mechanical stimulation (Leaõ, 1944), evoked by a few light touches on the exposed surface of the cortex with a glass rod. Mechanical stimulation of this form is insufficient to cause visible structural damage and need involve only slight compression of the neural tissue.

The application of potassium chloride (KCl) produces a rather similar effect to repeated stimulation or mechanical pressure and is the most commonly used technique.

Spreading cortical depression is a phenomenon of brain function which occurs in a number of mammalian species. There are, however, quite marked species differences. Spreading depression in an investigation by Von Harreveld, Stamm and Christensen (1956) was produced consistently in the rabbit, at six to ten minute intervals. A series of spreading depressions could be induced in the brain of the cat, but only using a longer interval (15 to 20 minutes) between stimulations. It was only rarely possible to obtain a series of depressions in the brain of the monkey even though long intervals were allowed between stimulations.

There is some evidence also that spreading cortical depression may be observed in older but not in younger animals. Laget and Neverlee (1963) found that it was impossible to elicit the response from infant rabbits before the age of 15 days. After this time, spreading cortical depression can be induced consistently, the amplitude relating to the steady cortical potential, growing from 3–4 millivolts at 15 days to 7–8 millivolts at one month of age.

Whilst spreading cortical depression may be reliably elicited from the rabbit and the rat, it is suggested that higher species in the normal state may have additional cortical systems which inhibit its consistent appearance. It is difficult to obtain evidence of its appearance within the human brain although Ochs (1966) reports spasmodic appearance in certain pathological conditions.

THEORETICAL VIEWS

Views about the mechanisms of spreading cortical depression fall into four main categories. First the theory that the cortex in showing cortical depression is in a dehydrated or pathological state, a view held by Marshall who believes that cortical depression may be produced only in the dehydrated cortex (Marshall *et al.*, 1950; Marshall and Essig, 1951). But this seems unlikely because spreading cortical depression has been produced in isolated pieces of cortical tissue bathed in fluid (Delisle Burns, 1958).

The second view is that of vasoconstriction. Leaõ (1947) observed vasodilation consequent upon the electrical wave of spreading cortical depression. Von Harreveld and Stamm (1952) point out that the vascular response to the phenomenon of spreading cortical depression is likely to take the form of constriction of the blood vessels. They are inclined to attribute the neural effects of spreading cortical depression to the vasoconstriction which appears to travel with it. Whilst the time relationships between the wave of cortical depression and that of vasoconstriction appear to be in phase, later work (Ochs, 1966) suggests that the vasoconstriction response accompanies cortical depression rather than acting as the means of its transmission.

The third view is that of transmission by electrical fields expressed by Sloan and Jasper (1950). It supposes that a slow potential discharge is the agent involved in cortical depression, and that electrical fields spread across areas of cortical tissue engulfing inactive neurones at the edge of the wave. This view has been criticized on a number of grounds, the most potent criticism being that a small incision of the cortex prevents the transmission of the wave. An electrical field should be unaffected by such an obstacle.

Von Harreveld *et al.* (1956) studied the transmission of spreading depression across a cut which severed all levels of the cortex. The preparations were allowed varying periods between three weeks and three months in order that healing could take place. In some cases the scar was less than 0.1 mm wide, but nonetheless an incision of this size was sufficient to act as an effective barrier. The fact that there was no transmission of spreading depression contradicts the view that a slow potential discharge is the agent responsible for propagation.

Grafstein (1956) challenged the electrical transmission view by placing cuts at different depths in the cortex. Whilst his results showed that conduction was carried out by no one layer of the cortex alone, cuts made through the upper parts of the cortex acted effectively to block the transmission of the wave. Monakhov *et al.* (1962) also showed that spreading cortical depression is not confined to the upper layers of the cortex, and the effect of incisions in impeding the progress of the depression wave has been demonstrated by other investigators. This work has cast doubt on the electrical transmission theory of cortical depression. It would be expected that electrical fields, if they exist, could easily bridge cuts and the fact that transmission does not take place across them appears to rule the theory out.

The fourth view is that of chemical transmission. Potassium chloride is used as the inducing agent. It is possible that the leakage of potassium from the finer processes of nervous tissue into the interstitial spaces is largely responsible for the massive depolarization of neurones, and that once induced, it sets off a chain reaction whereby other cells lose their potassium with further depolarization (Grafstein, 1956). Glutamic acid has also been suggested as a substance which, in its release from nerve cells, may be instrumental in transmitting the wave of spreading cortical depression (Van Harreveld, 1959).

Evidence is available which suggests that a swelling of apical dendrites takes place during cortical depression (Van Harreveld, 1958), and that during the passage of the wave, an entry of chloride ions occurs (Schadé, 1964; Van Harreveld, 1966). Ochs has suggested (1966) that not only are the internal constituents of the neurone released into the extracellular spaces (K+ and possibly glutamates), but also the dendrites, because of increased permeability, take up the sodium and chloride ions of the extracellular medium. Whilst the means of transmission of the wave of electrical activity is still somewhat controversial, there seems to be general agreement that transmission of depression across the cortex, leading as it does to a loss of cortical function, cannot be regarded as one of the adaptive functions of the brain. It appears as a general response to brain trauma and would seem not to be representative of normal function.

TECHNIQUES

The techniques for inducing spreading cortical depression have been described by a number of authors. One method is to make a midline incision in the scalp and to expose the brain surfaces of both hemispheres through bilaterally placed trephines. The scalp is secured with several temporary sutures. When spreading depression is to be administered the sutures are untied, the scalp is drawn back, and filter paper soaked in 25 per cent KCl is applied through the trephine hole to the membrane around the brain (Bureš, 1959). Russell and Ochs (1963) developed a more advanced system, whereby KCl-soaked cotton wool is placed on small plastic cups inserted into bilaterally placed trephined holes. Each cup has a hole which allows the solution to reach the dura. Schneider and Behar (1964) describe a modification of this technique in which the parietal brain surface of both hemispheres is exposed, but the scalp is sutured to a rubber grommet surrounding both trephines. This avoids repeated retraction and resuturing of the scalp.

Several authors have reviewed the literature on spreading cortical depression and for a more comprehensive account the reader is referred to the following: Delisle Burns, 1958; Marshall, 1959; Ochs, 1962. Our main concern is not with the finer detail of nerve function or with the details of technique, important though these are for an understanding of the phenomenon. Our concern is with the light which this technique has thrown upon the relationship which each hemisphere holds to the other in the control of function in the animal brain.

HEMISPHERE FUNCTION

The essential aspect of this technique is the temporary removal from function of one cerebral hemisphere, so that it is possible to state how the functioning hemisphere responds in the absence of its companion. It is also possible to investigate how information is transferred from one hemisphere to the other by first depressing one hemisphere during training, releasing it, and then depressing the other during test trials to establish the nature and the extent of information transfer. Using this method, we can compare the functions of each hemisphere one with the other.

As will be seen later, the results of this method provide a picture of brain function in animals whereby each hemisphere appears to be the identical twin or duplicate of the other. Each contains the necessary equipment to control behaviour even in the absence of its companion. Each shares the same characteristic stamp of the individual with regard to learning performance. Each has the capacity to perceive, to remember and to learn. In ordinary circumstances information is shared between the hemispheres, such that each corresponds in its stored experience to the other. The pattern which emerges as far as the functions of higher control are concerned, is of a duplicate brain in which the potential of each half is mirrored by the other.

LEARNING

Spreading cortical depression has been used to provide information about the relationship between hemisphere functioning, learning and remembering. Bureš (1959) applied spreading depression to one hemisphere, at the same time leaving the other free to carry out its usual function. He reported that rats have the capacity to learn a variety of tasks with only one functioning hemisphere and each appears to have equivalent capacity to the other. When the animals were trained using one hemisphere alone, clear retention of the task by that hemisphere was observed. When, however, the functions of this hemisphere were removed and the functions of the other released, no evidence could be detected of the transfer of learning from one hemisphere to the other. In fact the fresh hemisphere required an equivalent amount of training to reach the performance criterion. Bureš supposes therefore that under these circumstances learning occurs exclusively in the functioning hemisphere. Bureš and Burešová (1960) describe similar work and come to similar conclusions.

OPERANT BEHAVIOUR

Operant behaviour may also be used. Russell and Ochs (1960) trained rats to press a lever to obtain food. The animal learned this task during one-hour sessions with one hemisphere depressed, and took only a few days to establish its response. Learning was present only on the side which had remained active during training. When the active hemisphere was one and the same as that used for training, the animal showed high rates of response. When both hemispheres are functionally depressed, operant behaviour such as that shown in pressing a bar to avoid shock or to obtain positive reinforcement in the form of food, is also eliminated (Bureš et al., 1961; Olds and Travis, 1960).

One of the most powerful mechanisms for reward are those associated with the hypothalamus, described as the hypothalamic 'pleasure' areas. Rüdiger and Fifková (1963) arranged an experiment in which rats pressed a lever to receive electrical stimulation in this area. Unilateral spreading depression was employed. Its effect, as in other investigations, was equal and opposite across the hemispheres. If, however, the reward centre of the hypothalamus chosen for stimulation was on the same side as the hemisphere in which depression had been induced, response rates declined. This suggests that the reward centres of the hypothalamus are lateralized in function, and that the hypothalamic area relating to each hemisphere is responsible for the stamping in or rewarding of response specific to that hemisphere.

Whilst the hypothalamic systems are clearly associated with the subsequent rewarding effects in behaviour, the frontal areas of the brain usually have attributed to them a role as the organizer of response. The frontal areas of the cortex, for example, play an important part in the control of operant behaviour. Spreading cortical depression induced bilaterally in the frontal areas of the brain of the rabbit abolishes bar-pressing behaviour after a latency of only two minutes, whereas spreading depression induced in the occipital areas abolished it after a latency of five minutes (Suzuki and Uneoka, 1966). This not only points to the importance of the frontal areas, but also suggests a method of pinpointing the zones of control for particular responses.

In considering the part played by each of the cortical pair, it is clear that operant response can be carried out by one hemisphere alone

(Russell and Ochs, 1960). The single hemisphere is not, however, the equal of the tandem arrangement and some impairment is to be observed in solo performance (Suzuki and Uneoka, 1966). Motor interference may exist as the result of functional cortical ablation, but the fact remains that response is still extant when only the single hemisphere is functioning. Although the loss of its partner is not without some effect, each hemisphere is capable, independently of the other, of conducting and maintaining the complex sensory and response sequence of operant behaviour.

HABITUATION

Upon repeated exposure to particular stimuli, an animal may fail to make the response which it showed in the initial trials, and it is then said to be habituated. Nadel (1966) examined habituation by testing response to a plexiglas environment under bilateral and unilateral spreading depression. The activity of the animals was used as a measure of habituation. The association of habituation with cortical function is by no means as clearcut as with other forms of learning. In the first place all animals, whether operated on or not, whether exposed to cortical depression or not, were significantly more active at the beginning than at the end of each individual test session. The stimulus of being moved into the test environment may have been responsible for this. On the other hand, it could be as Nadel suggests, that it represents a form of short-term habituation controlled through subcortical regions. It was found that rats, operated on but not exposed to spreading depression, habituated to the situation and became less active, whereas those with unilateral spreading depression failed to show a loss of activity and those exposed to bilateral spreading depression in fact increased their activity over the six trials of the experiment.

Nadel suggests that the cortex is essential to the storage associated with permanent memory. The fact that animals with one cortex failed to show significant habituation although displaying a tendency in that direction could suggest that one hemisphere alone is not capable of carrying this out and that in the ordinary course of events both hemispheres take part in habituation.

There are two considerations to bear in mind in the interpretation of these results. In animal learning, the growth of performance may not simply reflect learning of the problem, but also learning not to be afraid (Dimond, 1970). The study by Nadel seems to be concerned as much with the diminution of fear as with the development of exploration, and as such relates to emotional behaviour. It could be aligned with studies of aversive learning which, as we shall see later, appear to involve subcortical mechanisms.

It is also possible, as Nadel himself points out, that we are witnessing not an inability to store permanent memory of the testing environment, but a marked interference with locomotor function through temporary cortical ablation.

Squire (1966) also studied 'habituation' during spreading cortical depression. Rats were placed in a T-maze and the number of turning movements by the animals was made the measure of habituation. This experiment showed that habituation can take place at least in respect of the turning response, even though depression may be switched to a previously intact hemisphere or applied again to a previously depressed one. This again suggests that subcortical structures are involved, and that information may show transit across the brain to be available to the untested hemisphere.

The fact that information becomes available to a hemisphere which at the time of transmission is in a state of functional ablation suggests that subcortical mechanisms provide a cross-communicating link. The fact that habituation does not take place under bilateral functional ablation suggests that the cortex carries out the necessary antedating analysis for habituation but that subcortical mechanisms, operating as a transport system, may lack the sophistication to carry out habituation itself.

A note of caution must be sounded, however, in interpreting the relationship between habituation and cortical function, because it is possible that a motor deficit consequent upon cortical depression will exert a marked effect on the results. Squire (1966) reported that rats showed a strong tendency to turn in the direction ipsilateral to the depressed hemisphere, and this again suggests that motor interference may play a part.

AVOIDANCE LEARNING

Some of the research has centred around avoidance learning. For instance, Bureš and Burešová (1960) carried out standard avoidance conditioning procedures on rats. The left hemisphere was functionally ablated by 25 per cent KCl solution. Next day, when the depression was switched to the right hemisphere and the left released, it was found that the same amount of training was needed to reach the criterion. In other words, there was no saving, and this was taken as evidence that the transfer of information about the task from one hemisphere to the other had not taken place.

Since the time of these original investigations (Bureš, 1959; Bureš and Burešová, 1960) appreciation has grown that the lateralization depends to a large extent upon the complexity of the task. In operant behaviour and in complex differentiation, information may be confined to the original hemisphere, but with regard to simple discriminations and those tasks which involve 'vegetative' or 'emotional' components, some transfer may occur. Bureš *et al.* (1964) themselves showed that passive avoidance conditioning established by the use of one hemisphere, may in part spread to the other despite the other's depressed condition. This is to some extent a reversal of the earlier findings. The suggestion arises that subcortical structures are more explicitly involved in avoidance learning than had formerly been supposed. It seems likely that these regions are concerned both with the transfer and storage of information concerned with the avoidance response (Bureš and Burešová, 1963; Kupfermann, 1966; Rabadeau, 1966). Transcortical transfer by means of subcortical mechanisms has been established in two further investigations. Schneider (1966) reported that rats trained to avoid shock under unilateral spreading depression required fewer trials to relearn the task when it was repeated under bilateral spreading depression. Kukleta (1966) also reports that many functionally decorticate animals retain the capacity for avoidance response after training under unilateral depression.

The studies of avoidance learning seem to suggest, in spite of the early studies, that significant transfer can take place even though cortical areas may be functionally ablated. This implies first an interchange of information between hemispheres although one may be functionally depressed, and second the presence of control stemming from the substitute areas of the subcortex.

MEMORY

By spreading cortical depression, it is possible to remove areas of cortex from function and determine if a given memory is present or not. One of the major findings has been that memory is not confined to a single hemisphere but exists in a duplicated and fully bilateral form. It is possible through experimental manipulation to implant one memory in one cerebral hemisphere, and at the same time, a totally different memory in the other. An experiment is reported in which rats learned a position discrimination whilst both hemispheres were intact (Bureš and Burešová, 1960). One of the hemispheres was then depressed and the animal was taught the opposite discrimination position. This opposite discrimination appeared in performance as long as the same hemisphere was depressed, but when depression was induced on the opposite side, the first position discrimination made its appearance. This shows that under special circumstances the hemispheres may be induced to store different kinds of information, and that information emanating from different hemispheres may establish different kinds of response.

The technique is frequently used to study the possible transfer of a learned engram from one hemisphere to another. Even when the hemispheres are allowed to resume normal function, spontaneous transfer of the information associated with a learning task may not always occur (Russell and Ochs, 1961). Rats were trained in an operant situation for one hour each day. One hemisphere was depressed whilst the other remained in a functional condition. The rat was required to press a lever to obtain a food reward. In spite of the fact that one hemisphere was depressed, the rat learned this task successfully after several training sessions. The necessary information for the task had become established in the functioning hemisphere. Each hemisphere is capable of systematic learning of operant behaviour on its own account, and each, admittedly under particular experimental conditions, can be trained to accept different memories from the other.

When, however, function is removed from the previously active cortex and invested with the other hemisphere, the animal shows no evidence whatsoever of having previously learned the task. Spontaneous transfer does not occur. This suggests a direct deposition of information as the result of learning in the one trained hemisphere.

The question now arises as to the speed of information transfer. Russell and Ochs (1961) suggested that in an operant training situation transfer may be effected on a single trial. This was supported by Bicens and Oakley (1965) who showed first that rats can be easily trained to make a brightness discrimination with one functional hemisphere; secondly that after release from functional ablation, a single trial is all that is necessary for information to transfer to the untrained hemisphere. The speed of transfer was tested by Kohn (1967) using a rearranged or fragmentary stimulus pattern. The animals learned a brightness discrimination whilst one hemisphere was functional. When a single trial was permitted during which neither hemisphere was depressed, a saving in new learning occurred which was roughly equivalent for both hemispheres indicating something of the rapidity of communication when the hemispheres resume their customary function. This work suggests something of the facility for information transfer between the hemispheres, which seem to be engaged in almost constant cross-talk. These results certainly point to powerful intercommunication links which keep each hemisphere informed of the functions of the other, and in transferring the details of stored memories, ensure that each retains the common experience of the individual.

Time relationships, in addition to the number of trials, are important in determining whether transfer will occur or not. Ray and Emley (1964) confirmed that transfer can occur on a single trial and showed that if only a short period of time is allowed to elapse, 15 seconds in this case, between the end of the trial and the onset of depression in the trained side, then transfer fails to occur. It is possible that information can be transmitted only gradually. If there are limits on the capacity of the cross-conduction systems, then stored information may have to queue before gaining access to the neocortical bridge. Alternatively, as Ray and Emley suggest, this finding is in line with the view that consolidation of the memory trace is necessary over a period of time before retention of learned material can take place.

As in avoidance learning, the situation is complicated by the possibility of subcortical involvement. The investigations do suggest that some sort of consolidation, perhaps of a more complex kind than we have hitherto thought, is necessary for the storage of information. This is shown by the fact that memory deficits for avoidance performance are obvious when spreading cortical depression is applied immediately after the training trials have been administered (Kupferman, 1965).

Schneider (1967, 1968) suggests thst the areas of memory storage may be displaced by spreading depression, from the cortex to the subcortical regions. The role of the subcortical regions is a complicating factor and it is certainly necessary to bear in mind that what might be interpreted as hemisphere ablation could represent little more than the blocking of functional areas of the major hemisphere and displacement to subcortical areas.

It is not the intention here to develop in detail the arguments which concern localization of memory functions. It is the purpose to show that the cortex of each hemisphere appears to show equivalence in the nature of its capacity for memory, and that although each may be made to learn or remember different things, the interference produced by cortical depression is roughly equivalent in its effect on both hemispheres.

INTEGRATION OF FUNCTION

The question we now have to consider takes us beyond that of functional equivalence. Spreading cortical depression has been used to unravel something of the relationship which one hemisphere bears to the other. In the case of bodily movement, in particular the movement displayed by the limbs, it would appear that control of motor output can be undertaken at the behest of either hemisphere, and that motor control can be interchanged between one hemisphere and the other.

Rats divide roughly equally into right and left hand groups on a task where they must reach through an aperture for food (Burešová *et al.*, 1958). But when they are forced to reach for food with their left forelimb, after denervation of the right, many of them subsequently remain left-handed. This procedure then entails a permanent change of preference. Either the original hemisphere still exercises control over the fresh limb by sending messages through the corpus callosum, or the change of limb is accompanied by a change of hemisphere. The former would suggest that each hemisphere not only manifests control over that side of the body to which it is *directly* linked through the precentral gyrus, but that it also has the capacity, if occasion demands, to control the opposite side by an *indirect* link, using the corpus callosum (Dimond, 1970b). In other words, one hemisphere may exert control over both sides of the body.

Inter-hemispheric integration has also been studied in the synthesis of memory traces (Burešová and Bureš, 1965). The work of Bureš and Burešová (1960), Russell and Ochs (1961), Travis (1964), Travis and Sparks (1963) may be quoted. They show that a duplicate set of memory traces is imprinted in one hemisphere by the action of the other. In normal function a close relationship must be maintained between the hemispheres, the memory material of one matching closely the memory material of the other. The question arises whether different memory traces implanted in each hemisphere may be combined to facilitate performance.

Burešová and Bureš (1965) established information of an escape reaction in the left hemisphere, by which the animal was required to jump on to a platform to avoid receiving an electric shock from a grid floor. At the same time information was established in the right hemisphere, of a conditioning task in which a buzzer sounded for a period of ten seconds, during the last five of which the animal received an electric shock from which it could not escape. When the animals were tested with both tasks combined, the sound of the buzzer was sufficient to ensure that they jumped on to the platform to avoid an electric shock. In fact the speed and efficiency with which the animals synthesized these two types of information, both we assume laid down in different hemispheres, was equivalent to the synthesis achieved by animals with reactions established within the same hemisphere.

There is some evidence to suggest that more efficient performance occurs when two hemispheres acquire different pieces of information than when both types of information have to be acquired by the same hemisphere. In this case two heads literally are better than one, in spite of the fact that information may have to be combined from different sources.

In a further experiment, Burešová *et al.* (1966) showed that the use of two hemispheres, with synthesis of information from both, produces better results in establishing an alternation reaction than the use of one hemisphere alone. Experimental animals were trained on a T maze using their left hemispheres. They were given electric shocks until they ran to one of the safe arms of the maze. On the next trial they received shocks until they ran to the opposite arm of the maze. When this alternation reaction was established, the animals learnt an escape task using only the right hemisphere, in which they received electric shocks until they jumped on to an elevated platform. They were then tested with the functions of both hemispheres intact, in an apparatus which combined the two forms of test previously described. Electric shock was avoided not by running through a maze, but by jumping on to one of two platforms, either to the right or to the left. This was not all, however, because successive trials involved alternation of response between one platform and the other. The results showed unequivocally that animals trained on the two component tasks using different hemispheres were superior to animals trained on the earlier tasks using only one hemisphere, and also those trained with both hemispheres intact on both of the tasks.

This important experiment shows that when sharing takes place between hemispheres, performance may be enhanced. Although each hemisphere has the capacity to learn and to remember, a double system may be very much better than a single one. It suggests too that the limits of intellectual capacity or information processing may be related to the joint action of both systems. Might it be the case then, if two systems are better than one in this experiment, that cooperative interaction is a customary mode of brain function in the normal course of events?

The finding suggests the idea of a reservoir for function which could be an integral part of the system. If one hemisphere is occupied with a particular task or taken up with the storage of certain types of material, then capacity may be maintained by the other which takes an additional load and thus extends the total capacity of the organism. The tandem hemispheric arrangement not only simplifies and facilitates performance, but may also extend the ability of the brain to sustain complex performances.

ALL OR NONE EFFECT

Spreading cortical depression has shown itself to be a valuable tool in the study of hemispheric function but there are certain points about the technique itself which need to be considered. First, it is important that the spread should occur in all or none fashion to avoid exposing the animal to stimuli connected with the learning task whilst the hemisphere is not completely depressed.

Bureš et al. (1962) describe spreading depression as an all or none affair occurring critically regardless of the stimulus values. However, Leaō (1944), Marshall (1959) and Tapp (1962) all suggest that spreading cortical depression occurs as a graded response, and Tapp (1962) suggests that the greater the concentration of KCl, the longer the duration of the effect. Cofoid (1965) measured the extent of spreading cortical depression by the use of bilateral electroencephalograms in rats. Analysis of the data revealed graded effects, with higher KCl concentrations (20 per cent) showing not only the longest recovery time but also greater amplitude changes. This question of the graded nature of the response complicates somewhat the value of the technique in the study of hemisphere function because the possibility of partial hemisphere function may have to be considered in circumstances where it would obviously be more convenient to state that the hemisphere fails to function at all.

More important than this, however, is the fact that depression appears to spread under certain conditions from the cortex of one hemisphere to the cortex of the other. Although it has been claimed that KCl elicits depression only in the hemisphere to which the substance has been applied (Bureš and Burešová, 1963; Tapp, 1962), some of the early observations suggest that in fact depression may be induced in its opposite number as well (Leaō, 1944; Leaō and Morrison, 1945).

Cortical depression showed no tendency to cross from one hemisphere to the other with weak stimulation, but as the strength of the stimulus increased, the depression of electrical activity in one hemisphere could be elicited similarly in the opposite one; the response appearing in the region symmetrically opposite to that stimulated but starting a little later. Stimulation of the frontal areas elicited a response from the opposite hemisphere more easily than that of regions further back. It was supposed (Leaō and Morrison, 1965) that crossed depressions involved the corpus callosum.

Stimulation of the underlying white matter after excision of the grey matter on one side produced symmetrical spreading depression in the opposite hemisphere. The hemispheres are linked by fibres which connect symmetrically opposite areas of the brain. Section of the corpus callosum prevented the transmission of depression from one hemisphere to the other (Leaō and Morrison, 1945).

Travis and Sparks (1963), Cofoid (1965), and Gollander and Ochs (1963) all report that the depression spreads from one hemisphere to the other although only one hemisphere may have received the application. Cofoid (1965) observed a clear transfer under the influence of 20 per cent KCl solution. If cortical spreading depression does extend its effects in this way, then the studies of hemisphere function are open to the objection that depression may have affected both hemispheres. This may explain something of the decrement in performance which is frequently observed. Where negative results are obtained, inter-hemispheric spread could be a factor, but it does not accord with the positive results of numerous experiments. Therefore it is not as serious an objection as it might at first seem.

MOTOR INTERFERENCE

Several authors have suggested that spreading cortical depression is associated with motor impairment (Thompson and Hjelle, 1965; Mogenson, 1965; Larsson, 1962). Tapp (1962), for example, reported a significant correlation between the loss of a conditioned avoidance habit and impaired sensorimotor coordination due to bilateral spreading depression. Delprato (1965) reports on the behaviour of rats tested in the open field situation under the influence presumably of bilateral depression. There was no evidence of changed emotional behaviour in terms of urination or voiding of faecal boli, but the animals were less active than the controls, crossing fewer of the lines of the open field. It is not clear if this results from diminished exploratory drive but what it could represent is impaired motor function. Change in locomotor activity raises serious problems for the investigation of functions such as learning and memory under the influence of spreading cortical depression.

The administration of KCl to only one hemisphere may reduce activity in a learning situation with the consequence that potential for learning is diminished. Comparison of learning performance of the treated animal with controls may not be justified, not because there are changes in learning capacity, but because locomotor activity may be different in the two cases. Failure to perform a task, attributed previously to the removal by spreading depression of a brain region, may instead be attributed to interference with motor activity. This possibility has been raised by Meyers and Stern (1968), who showed that the administration of bilateral depression reduces the amount of movement to a very low level indeed, and certainly to a level well below that of controls. Again this work points to the need for caution in interpreting deficits in performance as a failure of learning when they may instead reflect a diminished level of motor activity.

Winocur (1965) confirmed this in an ingenious way using two motor tasks of different levels of complexity. On one task rats avoided shock by entering a safe compartment through one of two open doorways. On another task they were required to locate a small centrally placed window and climb through it. Normal animals showed equal learning ability on both tasks. Rats suffering bilateral depression showed some impairment on the easy task, but also very bad performance on the difficult task which involved more complex motor skill.

Yet another difficulty has to be considered. We have seen that bilateral spreading depression interferes with motor behaviour. The suggestion arises that this is due to the influence of treatment on coordination. If it is acknowledged that there are bilateral effects, then are there unilateral effects also? Koppman (1963) describes the performance of rats in a two-way avoidance apparatus under the influence of unilateral depression. The animals showed a distinct tendency to turn away from the depressed side, so that the importance of the reward in determining their choice of direction may have been reduced as a result (Koppman and O'Kelly, 1966).

Rats reliably chose the side of the maze opposite to that of their depressed hemisphere. If this coincided with the reward, the rats scored nearly 100 per cent success on the very first day of the test. If, on the other hand, the reward did not correspond with the direction of choice, induced by the unilateral administration of KCl, then performance was extremely poor.

These experiments point to the need for complex controls to ensure that the observed effects represent something more than inferior performance through motor disturbance.

CONCLUSIONS

The difficulties associated with the use of spreading cortical depression must be discussed in any evaluation of the results. In many cases some measure of control has been exercised over the spread of the effect from one hemisphere to the other, and also over possible interference with motor behaviour. Further, the conclusions drawn on the basis of this work are often substantiated by investigations which employed different techniques.

The findings reported here indicate that each hemisphere is capable of functioning, in the absence of the other, as an information receiving, learning and remembering system. They emphasize the tandem construction of the brain and the essential dual nature of its functions.

However, while pointing to a surprising degree of equivalence in function between hemispheres, at least in the animals studied, these findings also suggest that the functions of each hemisphere are highly integrated one with another. Animals trained on two component tasks using different individual hemispheres may show performance superior to that of animals trained on only one hemisphere, or to that of normal animals trained on both tasks with both hemispheres. This suggests that two systems may be better than one and that the limits of intellectual capacity may be closely related to the joint action of both these hemispheric systems.

3

Hemisphere Disconnection
in Animals

INTRODUCTION

The corpus callosum is the largest cerebral commissure in mammals. Even in relatively primitive species it may contain many thousands of fibres. In man it forms a substantial neural structure and it has been estimated that it may contain as many as a million fibres (Bailey and Bonin, 1951). The corpus callosum increases in size and efficiency with ascent of the phyletic scale and one of the major advances in brain structure and organization has come about through the elaboration of rapidly conducting systems between one side of the brain and the other.

There has been much speculation about the corpus callosum, and experiments involving its division now provide a relatively clear picture of the part it plays in the organization of function within the brain. It had been clear previously from anatomical studies, too numerous to describe in detail, that a principle of homotopic organization applied to callosal distribution. The callosal fibres connect up symmetrical points on both sides of the brain. An area of brain on one side in one cerebral hemisphere is thus informed of the activities of the corresponding area of brain tissue on the other side. The corpus callosum thus acts as a coordinator of hemisphere function.

The corpus callosum was thought to exert certain types of fairly closely prescribed effects after Moruzzi (1939) had shown that the masticatory area of the rabbit was susceptible to facilitation by a barrage of impulses from the commissural region. At that time it was not clear whether these impulses exerted a general stimulating effect or whether they conveyed precise delimited information to the masticatory area.

The electrical response mediated by the corpus callosum bears out the homotopic projection of impulses between corresponding regions, and a number of electrophysiological studies show that electrical cross-talk is mediated by way of its fibres. Curtis and Bard (1939) and Curtis (1940a, b) analysed the electrical response of the neocortical

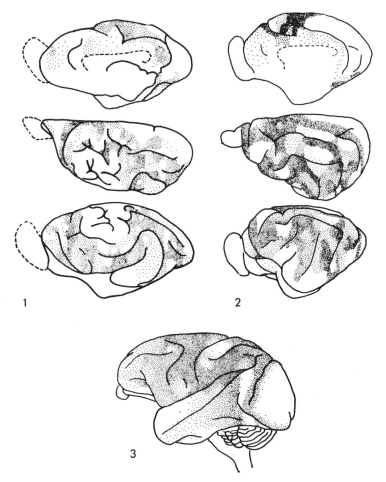

Fig. 8. Pattern of distribution of commissural fibres over the cortical surface of the left hemisphere of: 1. The raccoon. 2. The cat. 3. Macaca mulatta. (Myers, 1964. In *Functions of the Corpus Callosum*, edited by E. G. Ettlinger. London: J. & A. Churchill Ltd.)

areas of cats and monkeys to a volley of callosal impulses, and by this method were able to establish something of the density of the cross-lateral fibres and to verify the principle of homotopic projection. These early findings were later confirmed by using the strychnine neurononagraphic method (McCulloch *et al.*, 1941).

Chang (1953a, b) examined in detail the nature of the callosal response and showed that it was capable of interfering with the sensory response of the cortex. Although no evidence of facilitation was found, the convergence of the commissural pathways, and also those reaching the cortex directly through the thalamus, was demonstrated by the mutual blocking of both types of response.

Evidence of functional transmission confirms anatomical studies of widespread hemispheric linking through the cross-connecting fibres of the brain. Results also show that the effects are not all in the same direction. At times the fibres of the callosum may be used to facilitate these processes, at others they may be used to interfere with them. Whatever the nature of the effect, the responses testify to the importance of the callosal fibres in cross-linking one hemisphere to the other.

VISUAL TRANSFER

The corpus callosum plays a part in the transfer of many different types of visual information. Even in animals occupying a lowly position on the phyletic scale, it is clear that the mid-sagittal brain regions play a part in cross-integrating the functions of the bilateral brain. Muntz (1961), for example, was able to show that octopuses trained to discriminate between a horizontal and a vertical white rectangle using one eye will also make this discrimination when tested with the other eye. In other words, the information shows transfer from one eye to the other. There was, however, no transfer after removal of the fronto-vertical tract. Similar effects are observed in the transmission of visual information from one hemisphere to another in pigeons (Beritashvili and Chichinadze, 1939). Visual discriminations fail to cross from the trained to the untrained eye following section of the corpus callosum.

In discussing integration of information between one hemisphere and the other, we have to consider the optic chiasma, the point of crossing of the optic fibres, as well as the corpus callosum and other mid-brain commissures. The great optic tracts provide a cross-integrating system. Ascending contralateral pathways pass one another at the optic chiasma. The first task in a systematic investigation of cross-integrational systems within the brain is to section the optic chiasma. Visual input is now restricted from each eye to the corresponding ipsilateral hemisphere.

Myers (1957, 1962) reports experiments in which the optic chiasma was sectioned in cats. The cat with one eye masked receives visual information only to one half of its brain. The cats were taught visual pattern discrimination with one eye masked. They were then tested for their ability to carry out discriminations with the untrained eye. The animals learned to push on one of two doors of the correct pattern to obtain food reward. Normal cats showed a remarkably well developed perceptual capacity, being able to distinguish readily between closely similar stimuli. When chiasma-sectioned cats were studied, a marked deterioration in the capacity to make discriminations was observed. The animals showed a loss in visual acuity, but were able to make some discriminations. Furthermore, transfer of training from one hemisphere to another was possible, even if somewhat impaired.

That optic chiasma-sectioned cats trained with one eye can perform discrimination tasks using the other eye, reveals a high level of information transmission between the two halves of the brain (Myers, 1955). It also suggests that the areas of major transfer occur not at this level but deeper in the structure of the brain.

When the neocortical commissures were divided as well as the optic chiasma, the outcome was different. Information in this case failed to pass from one hemisphere to the other and subsequent relearning must take place, using the second untrained eye. As the number of available fibres in the corpus callosum diminished through the sectioning procedure in individual animals, so the degree of transfer declined. At first information about the more difficult problems failed to transfer, but as more of the callosum was removed transfer of the information for easier discriminations failed to occur.

Myers (1962) also showed that destruction of areas of a trained hemisphere as well as destruction of the corpus callosum result in a decrement in performance, again suggesting that a lack of information transfer is the key to the observed deficit. He showed that there is a much closer association in learning performance of an associative kind between the crossed and uncrossed visual interpretative mechanisms relating to a single hemisphere than between the uncrossed mechanisms of the two hemispheres connected through the corpus callosum.

The commissures appear to serve an essential role in the transfer of visual information from one half of the brain to the other and Sperry (1956) points out that there may be a characteristic imprint upon the learning processes of the hemispheres in a split-brain animal. The curves for the same individual will change on different problems but this variation tends to run in parallel. The fact that the two hemispheres show similar idiosyncrasies suggests that the nature of the learning curve is predetermined to a notable degree by the intrinsic functional organization of the cerebral hemisphere.

There is also some evidence that the memory trace in one hemisphere deteriorates, although the trace for the same task in the other hemisphere may be strengthened by additional training. Cats after section of the optic chiasma are taught to perform visual pattern discrimination with one eye masked. After overtraining, the corpus callosum and the anterior commissure are totally transected. Performance through the trained eye represents the degree of development of the memory-trace system within the one hemisphere and performance through the untrained eye the degree of development of the memory trace within the untrained hemisphere. Performances through the untrained hemisphere show a considerable deterioration following section of the commissure after training (Myers, 1959, 1961, 1962). The memory deficit in the untrained hemisphere relates to the difficulty of the task. Myers (1957) reports that recall of simpler tasks was good using the untrained eye, but poor or totally absent in the case of more difficult tasks. The outcome of this experiment was similar to that in which instead of section of the corpus callosum, critical parts of the trained hemisphere were removed. Callosal pathways may be passed over in preference for those pathways in the single hemisphere. If animals after section of the optic chiasma are trained subsequently to make a pattern discrimination through the left eye, and are then taught a second somewhat similar discrimination through the right eye, it might be thought that whichever eye was used, the most recently learned discrimination would be the one which occurred in preference to the other (Myers, 1964). This was not the case. When the animals were tested through the left eye they showed the original response trained through that eye. This again suggested that the type of training laid down was specific to a particular hemisphere and that the pathways leading to one hemisphere evoke responses within that hemisphere rather than those of the other side.

The neocortical commissures of primates appear to convey relatively greater amounts of information than do those of the cat. Inter-hemispheric transfer of a high order occurs in normal monkeys (Myers, 1964). Trevarthen (1962b, 1964) described investigations of the functional inter-relations in the split-brain monkey. Monkeys with chiasma and inter-hemispheric commissures sectioned were trained to work behind a fitted face mask with two eye holes which separated the visual paths of the two eyes. Looking through the mask the subject saw two small white plastic screens. The stimuli were projected on to these screens. The monkey to respond reached out and pushed one of the screens. Polarizing filters were inserted into the eye holes. One excluded vertically polarized light, the other horizontally polarized light. Projectors superimposed patterns on the screen. One projector was polarized vertically, the other horizontally. It was thus possible to present conflicting stimuli to the two eyes.

The first point to be noted about this work is that there were no emotional or other signs of conflict. Some of the responses were duplicated by both hands suggesting some loss of independent function. The evidence, however, pointed to the fact that two simultaneously conflicting memories of visual patterns associated with reward may be retained separately in the two halves of the cerebrum (Trevarthen, 1964). Sectioning of the inter-hemispheric commissures reveals two independent systems of visual perception, cognition and memory. Black and Myers (1964) report further on the relationship of the eye and the hand in monkeys with section of the corpus callosum. They were concerned with the way in which visual information is used to exercise manual control. They show that the inter-hemispheric transmission of visually guided latch-box solving skill in the chimpanzee is, to a very large extent, dependent on the presence of the forebrain commissures. The deficit in transfer was most marked following total section of the corpus callosum. It appeared clear from this work that section of the corpus callosum effectively blocks the transmission of certain types of information from one hemisphere to the other. Tasks involving complex discriminations may fail to transfer. There are, however, certain notable exceptions to this and some types of transfer occur which are not as yet clearly understood.

Very simple types of information were reported as crossing from one side of the brain to the other. Meikle and Sechzer (1960), for example, found that brightness or flicker frequency discriminations do show transfer of training between the eyes. Schrier and Sperry (1959) had suggested earlier that the transfer of brightness discrimination might be different from pattern discrimination. The animals studied by Meikle and Sechzer failed to show a transfer of pattern discrimination but each transferred the brightness discrimination at above criterion level. However, it appears that the transfer of simple forms of information occurs through forebrain commissures other than the corpus callosum. Meikle (1964) himself reported that if all the neocortical commissures were sectioned the transfer of brightness discrimination failed to occur and learning once again proceeds independently in the two hemispheres.

There are reports also that transfer occurs if an animal is trained in an aversive learning situation under shock motivation. Sechzer (1963) showed that pattern discrimination can transfer in the absence of the corpus callosum if cats are trained under shock-avoidance motivation. It is well known that aversive learning is one of the most powerful of techniques for establishing a response over the long term. This is also illustrated here in the capacity to bring about transfer from one hemisphere to the other. Aversive motivation may be able to exert the effects that it does and achieve correspondence across the midplane because of the implication of the pain mechanisms at the thalamic level.

Some of the generalizations about transfer have had to be qualified. The amount of transfer depends to some extent on the complexity of the task, the species studied and the conditions of motivation.

It is clear that the corpus callosum plays the principal part in the transfer of visual information, and this is substantiated in physiological studies. Hubel (1967) reported, using single cell recording, that of 34 single fibres recorded from the posterior corpus callosum, all but one or two could be driven by visual stimulation, and of these all but one had receptive fields that overlapped the vertical midline, or came up to within a degree or less of it. Fibres of the callosum could link cells whose fields lie close together on opposite sides of the vertical meridian. This suggests a function of immediate integration across the vertical midline. Many cells of the corpus callosum do show simple properties, but there are others which have complex and hypercomplex properties. The studies of Hubel support the view of visual transfer across the callosum. Recordings were made from a very closely circumscribed area and more extensive investigations of this kind are necessary over the wider area of the callosum to establish fully the nature of conduction functions.

The manner in which information is stored and transferred from one hemisphere to the other is of interest. In the unoperated pigeon, the optic fibres from each eye cross completely in the optic chiasma and terminate in the tectum of the opposite side of the brain. Mello (1965a, b) found that the unoperated pigeon showed interocular transfer but the mirror image rather than the original stimulus was chosen for response. It is possible that this happens because all features of the object are the same except those of its orientation. However, the mirror image is preferred over the original stimulus. This argues for topographical representation of spatial images which become reversed as the result of transit across the callosum and storage within the second hemisphere. Noble (1966) argued that reversal of this kind may be a generalized feature of inter-hemispheric transfer. The surviving optic nerve fibres from each eye pass only to the ipsilateral hemisphere in the monkey with its chiasma sectioned. If mirror image reversal is a feature of the transfer of visual information from one hemisphere to the other then the monkey also should choose the mirror image rather than the original training stimulus in a discrimination situation. Noble trained monkeys to discriminate between solid objects of different shapes. The non-mirror problem was solved correctly by the use of the untrained eye after original training. Similarly, where stimuli differed in an up-down direction, transfer was easily achieved. When, however, left-right mirror image stimuli were shown, the negative stimulus of the trained eye was treated almost invariably by that eye as though it were the positive stimulus. Mirror image responding appears to be a feature of the inter-hemispheric transfer of visual information. This points to the importance of left-right orientation not in any absolute sense of a relationship existing outside of the body schema, but rather in the construction of a sensory template specific to the eye. In other words, there is a clear imprint which has a distinct relationship to the eye. This imprint is reversed during transfer, thus preserving its topographical relationship.

ELECTRICAL ACTIVITY, SLEEP AND WAKEFULNESS

If the E.E.G. potentials are simultaneously recorded from symmetrical cortical points of the two hemispheres of the normal cat or monkey brain, they are similar in shape, amplitude and duration. The fibres of the corpus callosum act again as a cross-integrating system to preserve the nature of symmetrical response. The role of the corpus callosum in sustaining bilateral synchrony of the E.E.G. has been investigated by a number of authors (Claes, 1939; Bremer and Stoupel, 1956). Bremer (1958) reports that after section of the corpus callosum the E.E.G. spindles recorded from corresponding contralateral cortical sites of the *encéphale isolé* cat fail to show the usual bilateral symmetry and they are no longer in phase. Generally there exists a persistent lack of fine correspondence between simultaneous left and right electrical waves. Some authors report that bilateral symmetry is disrupted over a considerable period of time (Berlucchi, 1966; Magni *et al.*, 1960). Callosal section has also been reported to abolish the cortical after discharge in the hemisphere contralateral to that stimulated (Erickson, 1940). However, the question of electrical correspondence cannot be left there. Some authors report that there is little or no mismatching of simultaneous activity even following transection of the corpus callosum. Here we encounter difficulties in interpretation.

A quality of response such as symmetry is notoriously difficult to measure because the question has to be asked, how much in phase must the responses be in order that they can be described as symmetrical? Is it possible that small differences mean that the responses are no longer symmetrical? If different investigators employ different standards for symmetry then discrepancies about the results are highly probable.

De Lucchi *et al.* (1961) and Garoutte *et al.* (1961) present results at variance with those described earlier. They observed that the percentage of synchronous right and left side E.E.G. waves was not greatly affected by a mid-sagittal lesion through the corpus callosum and the massa intermedia of the thalamus.

Radulovacki *et al.* (1965) also reported that there is little if any difference between one side and the other in monkeys following section of the callosum, septum, massa intermedia, and anterior, habenular and posterior commissures. In cases of agenesis of the corpus callosum also bilateral synchrony of normal and pathological brain waves in human beings is a notable feature.

The hypothesis has been advanced by investigators who support the view that there is no major loss of synchrony following mid-brain division, that correspondence is maintained by the activity of a common pacemaker located in the brain stem. The corpus callosum according to this view forms at best only an ancillary pathway to the direct thalamo-cortical connections. This view is not without evidence to support it. It has been shown that bilateral E.E.G. asymmetries can be produced by unilateral brain stem lesions (Cordeau and Mancia, 1958; Rossi *et al.*, 1963). It is noteworthy, however, that the asymmetries which do exist consist of episodic mismatching between the change from synchronization to de-synchronization and vice versa associated with arousal or the advent of sleep. This is different from the lack of fine correspondence reported by Claes (1939) and by Bremer and Stoupel (1956).

Singer (1969) also reports that in cats with chronic electrode implantation and section of the corpus callosum, the anterior, posterior and habenular commissures, and the massa intermedia, there was no detectable loss of synchrony following section of the corpus callosum. There were differences between different regions of the same hemisphere, although these differences were again symmetrical across the brain. Section of the massa intermedia produced some dissociation of bilateral spindle activity and arousal response, but in all other conditions bilateral synchrony was maintained. Transfer of evoked potentials likewise was not influenced by the split-brain operation. Gazzaniga (1970a) has also shown that evoked potentials may remain unaffected in split-brain primates whilst at the same time stimulus information remains completely lateralized and confined to the single hemisphere.

These results, as well as those of after discharge (Straw and Mitchell, 1967) suggest that the corpus callosum, although important in other respects, plays only a limited part in coordinating the electrical rhythms of the brain.

The possibility has to be entertained in the light of studies on transfer of training after section of the corpus callosum that the patterning of E.E.G. waves is something additional to those imposed upon the cortical areas from the mid-brain region. Berlucchi (1966) whilst reporting that the normal bilateral symmetry is disrupted permanently by section of the corpus callosum, also reported that in the cat, the E.E.G. arousal reactions and onset of sleep patterns remain synchronous on the two sides. When lesions of the mid-brain are added to section of the cerebral commissures a mismatching of the waking and sleeping states of the two hemispheres is to be observed.

Thus it would appear that the correspondence between one hemisphere and the other, in respect of the patterns of sleep and wakefulness as manifested by the electrical activity of the brain, is controlled by the centres of the lower brain stem. Inter-hemispheric asynchrony of sleep as measured by the E.E.G. persisted over five months after callosal and midsagittal section.

Observations on monkeys suggest different results, however, and it is quite possible that phyletic changes could account for this difference. In the study by Batini *et al.* (1966) split-brain monkeys showed highly synchronized identical day-night rhythms as well as comparable periodicities. The patterns between the hemisphere of fine electrical activity including the simultaneous occurrence of spindle trains appeared unaltered in the split-brain animal. However, the ratio of sleep to wakefulness was sharply reduced. The percentage of time spent in wakefulness was found to be higher in the split-brain group. This result runs counter to the suggestion that the activities of one hemisphere transmitted through the other have an arousing effect upon performance and we must await further evidence before we can attribute a significant role to the corpus callosum in coordinating the patterns of sleep and wakefulness.

SOMESTHETIC SYSTEMS

The normal unoperated animal shows a high degree of transfer of somesthetic learning. Sperry (1958) reports that an animal trained to make a discrimination with one hand, of softness, weight or three-dimensional form is capable of showing the same discrimination when tested with the other hand. He argued that somesthetic discriminations along with the correlated motor learning transfers at a high level from the trained to the untrained hand. The question has to be asked as to what role the corpus callosum plays in effecting this transfer. Will animals with section of the corpus callosum fail to show such transfer? Stamm and Sperry (1957) suggest that although transfer occurs in some species it does not appear to do so in the cat. Cats were trained to push the correct one of two pedals. The cats could not see the pedals, which could be reached by one forepaw only. The animals were required to discriminate by touch alone with one paw on the basis of roughness, softness or form. They were then tested for transfer to the other paw. Animals with section of the corpus callosum, whilst showing facility for the learning of this task, failed to show transfer from one paw to the other.

A similar failure to transfer a learned tactile discrimination was reported by Ettlinger and Morton (1963). Rhesus monkeys were trained post-operatively to distinguish between two objects, a cylinder and a cube with one hand, the other hand being restrained. The animals were then tested for transfer. Only one of the five animals performed better than the level of chance. These results suggested that the callosum is involved in the transfer of learned shape discrimination. Semmes and Mishkin (1964) found in the chimpanzee that intermanual transfer of a learned unimanual skill was impaired following callosal section. Myers and Henson (1960) also report that whilst commissurotomized chimpanzees exhibited normal rates of learning with the first hand, they failed completely to solve the same problems with the other hand. Furthermore, failure of transfer extended not only to a failure to solve the problem but also to a failure to appreciate through their movements that there was a problem to be solved. A second box was manipulated as though it were the earlier problems presented to that same hand.

Kohn and Myers (1969) also reported that some of their animals failed to show intermanual transfer on a task in which thay were required to learn to open latch-boxes with one hand and were then tested for transfer with the other. Vision appears to be an important factor. Animals trained in the absence of vision required retraining using the other hand, and those trained with but tested without vision either refused to do the problem or required more time for its completion. Tasks of this kind are likely to require highly complex transformations. The corpus callosum plays a major part in the transfer of information associated with these complex skills.

Lee-Teng and Sperry (1966) looked at the problem of intermanual transfer on their experiment in which seven pigtail monkeys were trained to perform an intermanual size-discrimination task and were tested after split-brain surgery. In the first experiment the monkeys were required to pull the larger of two levers, one lever being presented to one hand, the other lever being presented to the other. In other words, they had to make a comparison of the relative size of the levers using one hand to touch each lever, and to pull the correct one, the larger of the two, to receive food reward. After the split-brain surgery the scores on this task fell rapidly to chance level. The authors state that cross-communication of manual stereognostic size information was eliminated.

Mark and Sperry (1968) trained monkeys to push a food item past an obstruction using one hand, the food dropped through a hole and the animal was required to catch it with the other hand. The dispenser was placed above a plexiglas sheet. the animal also placed one hand above this sheet and the other hand underneath. This task required that the animal use the sensory information for the direction, distance and timing of the target from cues originating in the other arm. The animals were trained using vision, and as soon as they had attained proficiency the forebrain commissures were sectioned. In subsequent training vision was not used. The greatest deficit occurred in the animal with the most extensive midline section. The lower hand was mislocated on numerous trials. This animal showed little improvement after the initial training. The defect in blind coordination was more severe than that when vision was permitted, but this showed limited improvement over time. In this experiment substantial impairments were produced by section of the additional mid-brain commissures although recovery of coordination over time shows that compensatory processes are possible through the use of other pathways.

In some investigations transfer occurred on some tests but not on others. Glickstein and Sperry (1960) trained monkeys to discriminate with either hand various different shaped or textured blocks. In the majority of tests section of the callosum effectively blocked transfer of the learned discrimination from one hand to the other. However, the behaviour of reaching out and feeling the test object transferred, although the specific pattern of finger movements used in testing failed to transfer. Nevertheless in a minority of tests there appeared to be some transfer of the specific sensory components of the habit.

Although certain components transfer from one hand to the other, it seems unlikely that this implies consistent transfer for other types of information by the use of extra-callosal pathways. There have been reports that, in respect of agility and muscular coordination, monkeys after section of the corpus callosum are hardly distinguishable from normal animals even after commissurotomies extending into the mid-brain region (Ettlinger and Morton, 1963). This suggests that there are important mechanisms of coordination in addition to the callosum. However, in the case of learned discriminations, failure to transfer represents a prominent feature of split-brain performance. The evidence clearly points to the importance of the corpus callosum in facilitating the information interchange about somesthetic learning between one hemisphere and the other.

EYE-HAND COORDINATION AND INTER-HEMISPHERIC TRANSFER

We have considered the transfer of tactually learned discriminations as well as the transfer of visual discrimination. The next task is to consider the part which the corpus callosum may play in integrating the motor functions with visual information.

Normal cats transfer information rapidly from one eye to the other on a task in which they are trained to displace a wooden block with the forelimb, and to discriminate between a black and a white block or one having a circle or a cross pattern. Discrimination of a pattern problem is achieved with the second eye in at least 82 per cent fewer trials than with the first eye (Schrier and Sperry, 1959). Following section of the forebrain commissures transfer of this kind may no longer be possible (Downer, 1959; Trevarthen, 1962b). Gazzaniga (1969) also reports evidence that bilateral transfer in respect of eye-hand coordinations fails to occur if the precaution is taken to limit proprioceptive feedback by restricting head movement.

There has been some challenge to the view that restriction of visual stimuli does not permit coordination of motor response by the opposite hemisphere. Bossom and Hamilton (1963) report in their studies of monkeys in which the optic chiasma, corpus callosum, anterior, posterior, hippocampal and habenular commissures were sectioned, that animals required to adapt to a prism worn over one eye show compensatory changes in the direction of movement which are a dominant feature of performance. Furthermore, these compensatory changes are not limited to one limb; the homolateral limb also displays adaptation to the same degree. This facility to adapt the performance of both limbs to altered visual input occurs in spite of the fact that the brain has been bisected. Hamilton (1967) also reports that little deficit could be observed in reaching behaviour when prisms were inserted in a mask over the animal's face and little deficit in transfer of the adaptation was to be observed when ipsilateral eye-hand pairs were used. Gazzaniga (1966a, b) had suggested previously that no cross-talk other than proprioceptive feedback may be necessary to explain ipsilateral eye-hand coordination in monkeys split down the mid-brain. He presumes that the arm governed by the blind hemisphere reaches to where the eyes and the head are directed. Thus the results of Hamilton could be explained on the basis of this view.

Gazzaniga (1969) restrained head movements by implanting steel screws into the skull of the monkey. A lightweight aluminium hat was fixed to these screws which connected to a Leitz ball and socket camera mount. Head movements were possible when this remained free, but were eliminated when the ball and socket joint was fixed. With the head free good contralateral and ipsilateral performances were observed on a lever-pressing discrimination task. With the head held, large deficits were seen in both the intact and the blind visual field. Gazzaniga argues that head and eye movements provide information to the hand which is used to direct it as at a target although no direct visual information reaches the non-seeing hemisphere. At the same time the possibility has to be entertained that this procedure interferes with postural mechanism and induces a deficit in transfer for this reason.

However, be that as it may, Gazzaniga's experiment throws interesting light on the problem of transfer and suggests a mechanism to explain apparent transfer effects in spite of the fact that the corpus callosum has been sectioned.

It points to the view that the corpus callosum plays its part in transfer and that there is a serious loss of performance after section, but at the same time one hemisphere can acquire knowledge of the functions of the other by the employment of proprioceptive feedback.

Gazzaniga's experiment suggests that in the absence of cross-cueing proprioceptive feedback, transfer fails to occur. It is noteworthy in this context that reports are common of the transfer of somesthetic discriminations, but reports on the transfer of visual discriminations not employing similar proprioceptive feedback are rare. This suggests that complex visual information cannot be cross-integrated whereas that employing proprioceptive feedback is. Gazzaniga (1969) suggests further that proprioceptive systems may provide cross-cueing mechanisms which, when removed from effective participation, leave the organism unable to cross-integrate the information in the ipsilateral eye-hand pair.

HEMISPHERE CAPACITY AND INTEGRATION OF FUNCTIONS

In studying the condition in which parts of the total information necessary for the solution of a problem are presented one to each separate hemisphere, investigations have been made of the integration of function. After indications that animals with section of the optic chiasma and the corpus callosum have been found to be able to learn an opposite discrimination habit with the second eye without any sign of confusion or retardation of learning (Myers, 1956), the question arose as to whether both hemispheres can learn separately but concurrently tasks which provide contradictory information.

The experiment of Trevarthen (1962) can be quoted again in this context. Polarizing filters placed over each eye of the split-brain monkey were used to separate visual input. The animal was required to distinguish between two patterns. One pair of patterns was polarized vertically, the other horizontally. One pattern of a given pair was rewarded throughout training for a specific eye, the other pattern being rewarded for the other eye. Learning was allowed to proceed with both eyes open until a reliable criterion had been attained. Each eye was then tested separately. The animals with optic chiasma, anterior and hippocampal commissures cut showed double learning. Both eyes retained the knowledge of the discrimination as though there had been simultaneous learning of the contradictory choice. No sign of interference between the rival learning processes was to be observed although the normal animal gave vent to considerable frustration when shown the two opposing stimuli. Something of this frustration and interference associated with conflicting pattern discriminations in normal monkeys was also observed in the split-brain animals in association with conflicting colour or brightness discriminations presented to the single hemisphere. The results suggest that in respect of more complex tasks which do imply separation, each hemisphere is able to proceed with the task independently of the functions of the other.

The problem of the integration of function was approached from a different standpoint by Sperry and Green (1964). They also employed polarized light filters which directed the information separately through each eye. The animals, to get reward, had to push the correct one of two illuminated panels. Right and left halves of the main stimulus figure were projected separately into opposite hemispheres. The problem could not be solved from the half figure information entering the single hemisphere alone. Normal monkeys or even monkeys with the chiasma sectioned but the callosum intact solved the problem easily. Monkeys with the corpus callosum sectioned were unable to integrate the information from both hemispheres and performance remained at chance level in spite of extensive attempts at retraining. Again when investigations were made to test integration the animals showed evidence that each hemisphere processed its information without knowledge of the functions of the other hemisphere. Evidence of independently adequate hemisphere function was shown when both halves of the information for the problem were projected to the single hemisphere. The monkeys were then able to perform at a high level.

Various strategies unrelated to the transfer of visual information can sometimes influence the results. Hamilton *et al.* (1968) took care to eliminate any possibility of this kind. These authors report that cross-comparison of coloured stimuli failed to occur in animals following complete section of the corpus callosum. With incomplete section there was evidence, however, of transfer occurring by way of the hippocampal commissure or the corpus callosum anterior to the splenium. The conclusion which these authors advance is that split-brain subjects are severely impaired on problems requiring inter-hemispheric integration of visual material. Although one monkey in their experiments continued to perform the cross-integrational task, this could be attributed to the fact that a band of unsectioned fibres remained by accident in the corpus callosum of this animal.

With certain noteworthy exceptions, it appears from studies of the integration of information presented separately to each hemisphere, that cross-connecting fibres of the corpus callosum play an important part. There is evidence from these studies that each hemisphere has the capacity to solve problems on its own even if at an impaired level when each receives all the necessary information. When information is distributed between the hemispheres, failure occurs pointing to a specific incapacity to unite the essential elements. There are some exceptions to this principle, however. Although complex elements may not be united, simple relationships can be established (Robinson and Voneida, 1964; Trevarthen, 1963). Gazzaniga (1966) also presents evidence that the activities of one hemisphere can be disrupted by action taken on information received by the other. Gazzaniga in studies of split-brain monkeys placed coloured filters over each eye. The animals performed a task in blue light, confining stimulation to the eye covered by the blue filter. Occasionally a red light was switched on which illuminated the contents of the cage. This was viewed through the red filter fixed over the other eye. If the monkey performed the discrimination task in blue light, and the red light suddenly illuminated the cage, the monkey was temporarily distracted but continued to respond as before. If, however, a toy snake were placed in the cage the blue-light task was abandoned and the monkey rushed to the back of the cage. This suggests that the activity of one hemisphere can disrupt ongoing functions of the other. It is possible that the controls became switched from one to the other as the nature of the emergency became apparent. This experiment is similar to those showing transfer in respect of emotional stimuli under spreading cortical depression. It suggests transfer of emergency responses at the thalamic level. In spite of these exceptions, as a general principle, animals are unable to solve problems unless the necessary elements are located in the single hemisphere. In the case of the projection of separate elements to each hemisphere, the animal with section of the forebrain commissures is unable to bring these elements into a meaningful relationship.

CONCLUSIONS

The split-brain animal is one in which the hemispheres show a functional separation so that each may be deprived of its customary knowledge of the other's function. Obvious impairments of transfer have been demonstrated. It is unnecessary to support the view that the functions of the hemispheres become totally divorced from each other, only to demonstrate that the transit of certain types of essential information is blocked.

Blocking is most easily seen on the more complex tasks. The importance of this fact is not diminished by investigations which show some residual transfer even in the absence of the mid-brain commissures. The proponents of the total separation view have sought to prove by experiment that various cueing processes operate which give the appearance of transfer although direct neural transmission is absent. The debate over this question need not concern us too greatly at the present time.

When information is lateralized to each separate hemisphere, not only may the hemispheres have the capacity to carry out conflicting discriminations (Trevarthen, 1962a) but overall brain capacity may be increased (Gazzaniga and Young, 1967). This leads to the view that the brain is an effective double system harnessed by the overall influences of the cerebral commissures, a view which is supported by the numerous studies outlined here. These show that no one hemisphere is totally deficient in performance, and that when information necessary for task performance is available to the single hemisphere, it is usually not beyond the powers of that hemisphere to perform the task. Each hemisphere therefore exerts considerable potential, and its separate performance is usually matched by that of its opposite number.

The normal brain of the advanced mammals, leaving aside consideration of the human brain, is a highly duplicate system in which the two halves give every appearance of working in parallel. The demonstration of an equivalent capacity within each hemisphere in the absence of the cerebral commissures suggests that the hemispheres of the animal brain may work in parallel for much of the time, although the possibility cannot be discounted that the functions of the hemispheres of the normal brain are closely integrated to extend the total capacity for performance.

4

Hemisphere Disconnection in Man

INTRODUCTION

The type of investigation which is used to study hemisphere function in animals pays close attention to the role of the corpus callosum as a transmitter of information from one half of the brain to the other. It has its parallels in the study of human brain functions, for which data have been gathered from a variety of sources. Principal amongst these are studies of callosal transection. However, evidence is also available from surgical studies following removal of a tumour, and from studies of patients in whom the corpus callosum has failed to develop, a condition described as agenesis.

Animal studies of hemisphere disconnection presuppose that no pathological brain process exists prior to surgery. In man though, callosal section is only performed if some accompanying brain pathology is already present and this often obscures a proper analysis of the results.

A variety of early reports exist in the literature. For instance, Liepmann and Maas (1907) describe effects on motor function. Trescher and Ford (1937) report the case of a patient in whom the posterior half of the corpus callosum was sectioned during the operative removal of a colloid cyst of the third ventricle. This patient suffered from internal hydrocephalus, and for several weeks after the operation experienced disorientation in space and a Korsakoff-like syndrome. He also had difficulty in naming objects and in reading words presented to the left visual field.

It is difficult in these early cases to determine exactly how much is the direct result of callosal transection. Dandy (1936) partially sectioned the corpus callosum for removal of pineal tumour and evacuation of a cyst of the cavum septi pellucidi and cavum vergae. He was unable to observe any mental changes following even extensive section of the callosum, and concluded: 'This simple experiment at once disposes of the extravagant claims to function.' It seems unlikely, however, that Dandy's techniques of psychological and behavioural measurement were sufficiently sophisticated to reveal any important differences which may have existed.

It was at one time suggested that the only demonstrated function for the corpus callosum was the transmission of epileptic seizures from one hemisphere to the other (McCulloch cited by Bremer *et al.*, 1956). It may be possible adopting this view to limit the spread of epileptic attack by section of the callosum whilst at the same time ensuring that little other damage occurs as a consequence of surgery. These reasons led Van Wagenan and Herren (1940) to section the callosum for the treatment of epileptic seizure. In some patients the corpus callosum was partially sectioned and in others it was completely sectioned.

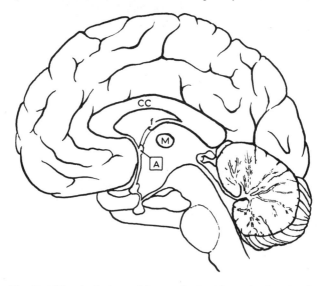

Fig. 9. Mid-sagittal view of human brain. The major interhemispheric communication systems are the corpus callosum (CC) and anterior commissure (A). Both of these structures are sectioned in patients operated on for surgical control of epileptic seizures. M, massa intermedia; f, fornix. (Adapted from *The Bisected Brain* by M. S. Gazzaniga, 1970. New York: Appleton-Century-Crofts.)

Akelaitis, in association with various collaborators, carried out an extensive series of case studies (Akelaitis, 1940, 1941a, b; Akelaitis *et al.*, 1942a, b; Akelaitis, 1944; Smith and Akelaitis, 1942). In addition to the dramatic observations that particular patients were still able to play the piano or touch-type with both hands there were also other systematic observations. These revealed that as far as ordinary behaviour is concerned there is little evidence of a deficit. For example, Akelaitis (1941a) describes investigation of visual perception. Disturbances of attention were not observed after surgery, and the patients were able easily to identify objects presented to the left or the right visual field. Perception of size and the recognition of colour in each hemisphere were shown to be impaired. Individual letters were recognized at the periphery of the visual field as easily after section of the corpus callosum as before. Furthermore patients were able to function with either homonymous field. Akelaitis suggests that each hemisphere possesses at least in a rudimentary form something of the mechanism for the visual aspects of language involved in reading.

A surprising observation was that colours as well as images could be fused stereoscopically, and this suggested that the corpus callosum played a distinctly limited part in the integration of information between the two hemispheres. Akelaitis himself regards these observations as furnishing no support for the view that the corpus callosum is of overriding significance, or support for the theory that a unilateral cerebral dominance exists in the evaluation of visual perceptions.

Further observations (Akelaitis et al., 1942) were devoted to a study of motor functions. Some patients were excluded because they showed a marked hemiplegia, the rest were subject to a variety of tests including studies on lateral preference which examined the dominance of eye, hand, and foot, as well as handedness of members of the patient's family (Smith and Akelaitis, 1942). The ability to handle objects as well as to execute spontaneous and imitative movements was also tested. The patients were required to carry out two activities at the same time, for example, to write with one hand whilst at the same time dealing cards with the other.

Some showed evidence of damage to motor systems before surgery; others showed post-operative damage. In ten cases motor functions were normal both before and after surgery. In these, three with complete section and seven with partial section, there was no evidence of dyspraxia and lateral preference remained largely unaffected. The patients could handle objects and execute spontaneous and imitative movements without difficulty. Two tasks were performed at the same time at a level which did not differ from performance prior to surgery. It might be argued that in selecting patients with no obvious motor deficit and in assigning them to a special group, Akelaitis had predetermined the nature of his results, i.e. he had selected out those patients without gross motor impairment. Nonetheless, deficits could well have been expected. Akelaitis argues consequently that dyspraxia in either hand after partial or complete section of the corpus callosum occurs only when damage to the subordinate or dominant hemisphere coexists with it.

Akelaitis et al. (1942) also comment on concepts of cerebral dominance and the light which their work throws on these and that the so-called minor hemisphere is capable of aspects of visual perception, and also that it can take on the functions of speech. Here it should be noted that by this is meant the capacity to read simple words and letters. They suggest that the subordinate hemisphere appears to be capable of reaching a higher state of development than had formerly been supposed. They also state that the idea that unilateral dominance is variable among different persons is an idea which even at that time was gaining ground. They imply that in some patients the dominance of one hemisphere over the other may be reduced. They also suggest that the relative youthfulness of their patients could explain the equipotentiality of function. In children, dominance associated with speech may be transferred to the subordinate hemisphere following damage to the dominant one, but this is unlikely as an explanation of these results, because all the patients, although some were youthful, were all beyond the age at which such transfer is supposed to occur.

Akelaitis pointed out the existence of other cross-connecting fibres in addition to the corpus callosum. However, he regarded the participation of these as improbable in view of their relative size and by virtue of the fact that finely synchronous coordination is achieved in such activities as playing the piano and typing. He supposed therefore that coordination following surgery is established by subcortical pathways.

The results so far suggest that the corpus callosum plays only a limited if any part in the integration of information from one side of the brain with that of the other. The studies, however, indicate the possibility of considerable bilateral representation in which the activities of one hemisphere appear largely parallel to those of the other. The degree of integration achieved by the hands in complex activities suggest also that as far as motor activity is concerned each hemisphere may exercise some control over the limbs on both sides of the body. Penfield and Boldrey (1937), as the result of cortical stimulation in more than a hundred cases, considered that ipsilateral response practically does not exist for motor movements. However, other workers have reported differently. Kennard and Watts (1934) were able to elicit ipsilateral movements by stimulation of the Area 6 of Brodman even after complete section of the corpus callosum. Bucy and Fulton (1933) also refer to clinical material which they believed was suggestive of ipsilateral motor representation in the motor cortex of man. Foerster (1936) in considering stimulation of the leg area in cases of internal hydrocephalus elicited movements in the ipsilateral leg both before and after section of the callosum. This suggests that each hemisphere may have embodied within it the potential to call out the motor movements of both sides of the body.

Following these early investigations, it is not surprising that the view became widely accepted that no important behavioural symptoms were to be seen in man following section of the corpus callosum providing that other symptoms of brain damage are absent (Akelaitis, 1944). Evidence of the lack of effect of callosal section must have been mainly responsible for leading Lashley to express his much quoted view that the corpus callosum has no other functional significance than to act as a physical support for the cerebral hemispheres.

As we have already seen, the impetus for further study came from work on animals, principally cats and monkeys. This led to a re-examination of the effects of section of the corpus callosum in human beings. Bogen and Vogel in 1962 describe how they sectioned the corpus callosum to treat a patient who had been having seizures for more than ten years, and who had continued to worsen despite extensive medication. Episodes of recurring seizures (status epilepticus) were present at two- to three-month intervals. Surgery involved retraction of the hemispheres and section of the callosum. Following this a considerable improvement was observed. It was reported that the patient had not had a single generalized convulsion over the last five and a half years of surgery, that the level of medication had been reduced, and that it had been possible to obtain an overall improvement in the patient's behaviour and well-being.

The second patient, a housewife and mother in her thirties, had similarly suffered severe and progressive attacks of epilepsy. The brain of this patient looked and felt normal. The corpus callosum and hippocampal commissure were divided separately. The other commissures were severed with minimal lateral trauma. At a period of four hours after surgery the patient could grip with her right hand and showed the Babinski reflex in her right foot, but at that time the entire left side remained flaccid, although she used both hands to pull the bedcovers over her. By the fourth week she was walking well although still apraxic with the left hand. By the eighth week, however, she had acquired good voluntary use of the left hand.

On the first day after surgery she showed some mumbling speech. On the second day she spoke intelligibly, and on the third day she was oriented in space, although at this time she did not recognize her husband. She remained disoriented with regard to time for the next few weeks, and difficulty in the recall of events persisted for many weeks. This patient also had remained free of seizures since recovery from surgery, and showed a return to the normal pattern of the electrical activity of the brain as measured by the E.E.G. (Bogen, Fisher and Vogel, 1965).

Sperry and his associates began an extensive study of these patients. A basic disconnection syndrome had seemingly been demonstrated in animals and the question arose as to whether this could also be demonstrated in man. Sperry (1968) stated that the symptoms in fact were not only present but grossly exaggerated. The first patient of Bogen and Vogel was found consequent to surgery to be unable to point with one hand to a spot which had been touched on the other side of the body, nor could this patient trace with one hand simple visual forms seen across the midline of the visual field. The left hand could not be used to write or to execute simple verbal commands. This patient seemed to represent the classical disconnection syndrome. If the brain is bisected in man then, as in animals, cross-talk between the hemispheres is disrupted. Geschwind and Kaplan had earlier identified a disconnection syndrome in a patient with a tumour involving the frontal and mid-sections of the callosum (Kaplan *et al.*, 1961; Geschwind and Kaplan, 1962a), and it appeared that the same syndrome was in evidence here.

The demonstration of the effects of hemisphere disconnection cast doubts upon the earlier conclusions advanced by Akelaitis that the callosum appears to play only a small part if any in the transmission of information from one cerebral hemisphere to the other. In the patients now described by Bogen and Vogel, the preservation of this structure appeared to be essential to the integration of hemisphere function. Without it the brain appeared 'as two individuals inhabiting the same body'.

Compensation may occur over time for the effects of section of the mid-brain commissures. This is particularly so with younger patients, and Sperry (1968) is inclined to attribute the fact that Akelaitis failed to report the human disconnection symptoms to the improvement which can take place in cross-integrational tasks shortly after surgery. He notes that the Akelaitis patients were sectioned in at least two successive operations allowing time between operations for at least some functional improvement to take place.

However, the evidence does not rest there. It has to be remembered that surgery is employed only after a severe and disabling illness and this can leave persistent functional defects. Secondly, the patients were epileptics who presumably retained the potential for seizure within one part of the brain, although the seizures themselves had been suppressed. The results are subject to considerations other than those pertaining to section of the callosum, and evidence obtained from a few cases, however dramatic, may still be subject to other factors.

In the more recent investigations conducted by Sperry and his associates, some features of the patients' behaviour run counter to those observed earlier. Some, for example, were able to localize cutaneous stimuli and to trace visual shapes across the vertical midline. Some could carry out verbal commands and write with the left hand and draw using one hand an object held out of sight in the other hand.

This contradicts the view that one hand has no knowledge of the functions of the other, and with more extensive observations the balance of evidence appears to have moved more in the direction if not to the same position as the views advanced by Akelaitis. However, it is still possibly too early to arrive at an adequate consensus because the quantity of the evidence even now is strictly limited, and the story is still a developing one. Reference is frequently made to the right or the left hemisphere here in the text. In order to avoid confusion in this and the succeeding chapters we refer exclusively to right or left function in the right lateral person. Exceptions are pointed out in the text as they become relevant.

AGENESIS

One of the curious facts about brain development is that on occasions the corpus callosum may be absent. The anatomical structure itself fails to develop and this condition is described as agenesis. It is a rare condition amongst the general population. Grogno (1968) reports that from London Hospital post-mortem records, only one case was found in 19,000 examinations. This occurred in a still-born infant having other abnormalities of the nervous system. Agenesis is more frequent amongst patients attending centres where the air-encephalogram is performed as a common diagnostic procedure. Carpenter and Drukemiller (1953) reported the incidence as approximately 3 in each 1,000 patients examined by these means. Grogno (1968) reports the diagnosis of 45 cases of agenesis amongst 6,450 encephalograms giving an incidence of 0.7 per cent. This suggests, as is indeed the case, that where agenesis occurs it is not uncommonly associated with other neurological abnormalities, although cases are reported in which this condition was unsuspected until revealed at post-mortem.

Cases occur spontaneously in the population but there is some evidence of a hereditary familial disposition in this as well as other associated central nervous system anomalies (Cozzi, 1963; Menkes *et al.*, 1964; Naiman and Fraser, 1955).

Developmental arrest which is responsible occurs during the first few months of pregnancy. The earliest fibres of the corpus callosum can be seen at 74 days of foetal life. The genu and the splenium, parts of the corpus callosum, are recognizable at 84 days, and adult morphology is attained at 115 days (Tilney, 1938; Ariëns Kapers *et al.*, 1960). Hyndman and Penfield (1937) report that the first evidence of the corpus callosum in the human foetus is to be found during the third month of development as a thickening of the lamina terminalis just dorsal to the anterior commissure. The most anterior portion develops first and its posterior enlargement leads directly to the formation of the septum pellucidum and hippocampal commissures. The earliest fibres lie anteriorly to the foramen of Munro. Subsequent fibres predominate superiorly and caudally producing the typical crescent shape of the adult structure. The developmental arrest of these systems can occur at any stage.

The early investigators were forced to rely on cases which had been discovered at post-mortem and in much of the early literature there is a considerable diversity of opinion. Bruce as early as 1889 expressed the view 'that if the brain is otherwise well developed, absence of the corpus callosum does not necessarily produce any disturbance of motility, coordination, general or special sensibility, reflexes, speech or intelligence'. Cameron and Nicholls (1921) also remarked 'that such meagre evidence as we possess seems to indicate that the callosal fibres are of much more importance in maintaining and governing the finer coordinations of muscular movement in the limbs of the opposite sides than in regulating the higher functions of mentality'. Hyndman and Penfield (1937), on the other hand, had reported that cases of complete agenesis of the corpus callosum were grossly defective. They report observations on five patients. Their general conclusion was that the patients diagnosed as complete agenesis showed gross developmental deficits, whilst in those diagnosed as partial agenesis no abnormalities were detected. For example, a 21-year-old man with partial absence but some residual callosum, obtained a rating of average on an intelligence test scale, and was able to comprehend and read written material with reasonable facility. A number of reports, however, suggest that the intellectual range of patients tends to be restricted (Koch and Doyle, 1957; Roone and Williams, 1962; Cozzi, 1963; Mueller, 1963; Nobler et al., 1963; Gyepes and Gannon, 1963; Menkes et al., 1964).

Although deficits in intellectual functions are common it must at the same time be said that there are cases where the person shows average ability and some above average ability. Patients of this type have been studied in detail, presumably because of their ability to cooperate with the experimenter and because of the interest in investigating patients whose intellectual performance is not depressed by other complicating factors. This became possible since the report of Davidoff and Dyke (1934) that air-encephalography can be used to diagnose agenesis in life. The classical features are dorsal extension and dilation of the third ventricle, wide separation of the lateral ventricles with angular dorsal margins, and dilated posterior horns.

Geschwind and Kaplan (1962a) describe a patient with atrophy of two-thirds of the corpus callosum. This was secondary to a circulatory impairment due to a cerebral neoplasm. The patient was unable to write with the left hand. He also identified objects incorrectly when they were placed in the left hand. Geschwind and Kaplan regarded this as an example of disconnection whereby the identification mechanism used by the left hand became separated from the language mechanisms in the right hemisphere. Russell and Reitan (1955) also investigated the behaviour of a 19-year-old woman patient who showed impaired visuo-motor coordination and inability to sustain concentrated attention. One feature of this patient was a marked deficiency of bilateral transfer of learning from the dominant to the non-dominant hand.

Jeeves (1965) also investigated the functional lateral relationships in agenesis. He employed tasks which involved integration of the activities of the hands. He studied 12 cases in all of complete or partial agenesis and points out that it is important to study cases with no other or at least with strictly limited additional cerebral anomalies. Jeeves describes a patient who, although showing an enlarged skull, appeared to have normal brain development apart from the agenesis. This patient was of borderline dull average intelligence. His verbal I.Q. was 84, his performance I.Q. 71. Jeeves reports that his motor coordination was equivalent to that of children ,of his own age, although he was somewhat slower in comparable tasks than normal subjects. The patient reads well, although he is somewhat poor at writing. He was compared with other children in respect of performance on psychomotor tasks. These were 'buttoning up', the pieces of the Merrill-Palmer scale had to be buttoned together. 'Winding string', the patient was required to wind a piece of string around a pencil, and a 'pegboard task', the patient was required to fit pegs into their appropriate places in the board. The patient performed these tasks more slowly than normal controls. This patient, whilst not demonstrating any marked impairment in general motor function, showed deterioration nonetheless on rather sensitive tests.

The possibility exists that subcortical pathways may play a part in the coordination of activities in the absence of the callosum. If the latter has never existed the use of other pathways would seem to be inevitable. Compensatory processes play a part from the earliest stages of development. Rutledge and Kennedy (1960) found in electrophysiological studies that in addition to the callosal response, an extra callosal response appeared after stimulation. It differed from the latter in several respects; in the first place it was delayed, but it was also weak and less stable. In all likelihood, the pathway of this may be used to compensate and Jeeves (1965) suggests that because there is an increase in contralateral response times in reaction time studies this implicates a devious route.

The case of a 14-year-old boy who scored within the normal range of intelligence was studied by Solursh et al. (1965). This patient's I.Q. was

107, verbal 95 and performance 115. He was given a variety of tests employing each hand separately or using both hands together. He was tested for the transfer of training to one hand after the opportunity to practise the task with the other. Generally he was able to identify objects and respond well using either hand, but difficulty was experienced in the integration of information across the midline of the body. For example, the patient was not able to tap correctly with one hand the same number of times that he himself had been tapped on the other hand.

The patient's performance on auditory tasks was perfectly normal, and he could perform commands with either arm to verbal instructions. With regard to visual perception, a very different picture existed. The patient was made to wear polarized glasses which directed the image only to the right or the left of the visual field. He was shown various designs. He could identify designs at the left visual field with his left hand, and he was able to identify designs at the right visual field with his right hand, but he could not identify designs with his right hand presented to the left visual field, nor could he identify with his left hand designs presented to the right visual field. In other words, the information necessary for this task was failing to transfer. Similarly, the patient identified many more letters when these were flashed to the same side as the hand used to identify them by writing.

This subject was tested for the transfer of learned information. In normal people information learnt through one eye is available when testing with the other eye. A series of five paired associate nonsense syllables were presented to the right eye from the right and learned by the standard anticipation method. The patient was instructed to write them down with the left hand. The series were then transferred to the left eye, and the patient was still able to perform the learned task perfectly well. It would appear from this result that in spite of the difficulty of identifying visual patterns with the opposite hand, transfer of learning is possible, but it may be that the investigation is not strictly comparable to animal studies of transfer of training because there is no reason to suspect that the cross-over point of the optic chiasma is disturbed, although the corpus callosum may be absent. There is, however, some evidence of impairment in the transfer of meaningful verbal material. The patient was shown five words to one eye, each of which belonged to the same family. Then a group of four words, one of which belonged to the same family, was shown to the other eye and the task was to identify the correct word. Some deficit in performance was observed, the patient identifying correctly 70 per cent of the words, whereas normal controls identified 100 per cent.

The results are somewhat equivocal in that there is evidence of a failure to transfer information from one side of the brain to the other in the case of visual patterns and complex generalizations, but in other respects transfer occurs as in a normal person. It is possible that extra-callosal pathways may be limited in their capacity to handle complex information, and that whilst compensation can be made for the absence of a corpus callosum, complete substitution with other mechanisms may not occur in its entirety and some deficit of a permanent kind remains.

Saul and Sperry (1968) point out that section of the neocortical commissures in man produced behavioural and neurological symptoms which require the implementation of special cross-integration tasks for their diagnosis. They investigated a case of agenesis to compare the effects of callosal deprivation on the one hand with developmental anomaly on the other. The patient was a 20-year-old college student in whom the entire corpus callosum was absent. This patient was treated after the development of acute hydrocephalus which gave rise to headaches. In an intelligence test administered before surgery, she was shown to be average or somewhat above average. Thus she represents a rare although not a unique condition. This patient is left handed and somewhat ambidextrous, a finding which Saul and Sperry describe as common among patients with agenesis. She had no difficulty in describing verbally material presented to either side of the visual field. She can easily identify objects placed in either hand and she had no difficulty in retrieving with the right hand objects similar to those identified by the left hand shown to the left visual field. If pairs of numbers were presented one to each half field, or if plastic numbers were placed, one in one hand, one in the other, the patient responded with the sum or the product as quickly as a normal person, showing that she had no difficulty in integrating the right and the left visual input.

The patient described by Saul and Sperry appears to be able to compensate for the lack of the normal integrating channel. Saul and Sperry note that the anterior commissure in this patient is enlarged up to one and a half times its normal size. Reeves and Carville (1938) also commented that enlargement of the anterior commissure may be a feature associated with agenesis and it is possible that this could facilitate cross-integration. It may also be possible that a patient of this kind develops strategies through self-education to improve integration of right and left functions in spite of the difficulties which are experienced.

The question now arises as to what can be concluded from these studies. Some degree of mental enfeeblement is present in the vast majority of cases. Different opinions exist as to the cause of the enfeeblement. Some authors suggest that the deficit can be attributed to associated anomalies (Kirschbaum, 1947; Loeser and Alvard, 1968) but it is by no means clear that the absence of the callosum does not bring with it an enfeeblement in its own right. Most cases show some impairment of mental function, and few cases score in the average range of intelligence and only the rare and exceptional scores above average. This suggests that in the early stages of development the absence of the callosum places the individual at a disadvantage for which it is difficult subsequently to compensate. The condition does depress intellectual function and the employment of subsidiary pathways cannot totally compensate for this disadvantage.

The presence of cross-integrational deficits is also another prominent feature. Geschwind and Kaplan (1962) suggest that lesion of the corpus callosum disconnects important brain areas from others. Something of this disconnection is evident in agenesis and it appears that in most cases reorganization of brain function to use alternative pathways never fully compensates for the loss of the most effective pathway.

CALLOSAL SECTION

In spite of earlier studies which appeared to attribute little if any function of significance to the corpus callosum, recent study suggests there are definable effects following transection. It has been said that transection disconnects one hemisphere from another. The use of the term disconnection may exaggerate the extent to which one hemisphere is in fact separated from the other and all links may not be severed. Even ardent supporters of the concept of disconnection may not wish to argue for a total separation of function. Some types of information do fail to transfer, but it seems probable also that direct neural contact is maintained for others through alternative routes.

We can regard section of the corpus callosum as disrupting important communication links and interfering with the transit of information, without the supposition of total cerebral disconnection. Where the term disconnection is employed it is used here to mean the disruption of communication patterns in the cross-talk between the hemispheres, and it is not the intention to imply a total neural separation between one hemisphere and another.

MOTOR FUNCTION

The first case of those reported by Bogen and Vogel seemed to follow the pattern of the callosal disconnection syndrome very closely indeed. When the patient was required to point with his right hand to a source of stimulation applied to the right side of the body, he was able to do so without difficulty. Similarly, he could indicate the point at which he had been touched on the left side of the body with his left

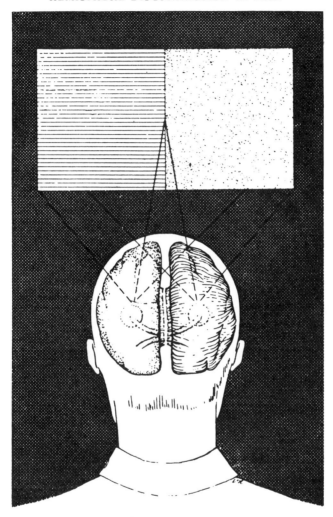

Fig. 10. The left and right visual fields of man are projected to the right and left hemispheres respectively. With the eyes held at fixation, crisp projection of information to one side of the brain or the other is easily possible. (From *The Bisected Brain* by M. S. Gazzaniga, 1970. New York: Appleton-Century-Crofts.)

hand. When given a choice, the patient almost invariably chose to use the left hand for stimuli on the left side of the body, and the right hand for points on the right side of the body. Some difficulty was experienced in eliminating auditory and other cues used in cross-localization, but when this was done the patient became inept at cross-localizing points with one hand stimulated at the opposite side of the body (Gazzaniga et al., 1963).

In a second testing session the patient was tapped at various points on the body one to four times according to a random schedule. The patient was requested to respond by tapping the corresponding number of times with his fingers on the palm of his hand. The difficulty experienced in cross-lateralization again became only too apparent. The patient could tap the correct number of times if the hand used and the place stimulated were on the same side. If the opposite hand was used the patient was unable to carry out this task. With regard to the senses of bodily position and pain and temperature, the same picture emerges. Points of cutaneous stimulation could not be located across the midline and information about somatic functions failed to transfer.

Gazzaniga, Bogen and Sperry (1965) describe further testing procedures. The patients were shown a bright spot of light ½ in. in diameter flashed in different areas of the visual field. The subject was required to point quickly to the spot where he had seen the light. When the stimulus fell in the right visual field it could be localized only with the right hand or verbally. Stimuli in the left field could be located only with the left hand and not verbally. When both hands were left free the first patient always used the right hand to point to stimuli in the right visual field and his left hand to point to stimuli in the left field. When one hand pointed the other usually remained motionless. Earlier indications that the left hand might at times respond to stimuli in the right field were not confirmed. The patient was shown a figure flashed tachistoscopically on the screen (Gazzaniga, 1970). He was required to select a similar figure from a group of five cards placed in front of him. The right hand usually responded correctly to patterns flashed to the right visual field. The left hand similarly responded although not as well to patterns flashed to the left visual field. However, the performance of both hands declined markedly when the information was flashed to the opposite visual half-field. In cases where stimuli were presented to the left field only, the subject would commonly deny having seen anything at all, and would be puzzled when questioned about what he had seen (Gazzaniga, et al., 1963).

Gazzaniga et al. (1965) report, however, that their second case, whilst demonstrating some of the features of the first case, was able to indicate using either hand points of stimulation on the body surface whether or not they occurred on the same or a different side as the hand. The most marked difference between the first and the second case was the ability of this patient to use either hand in responding to signals directed to the opposite hemisphere, or, for that matter, to use either hand in responding to verbal instructions.

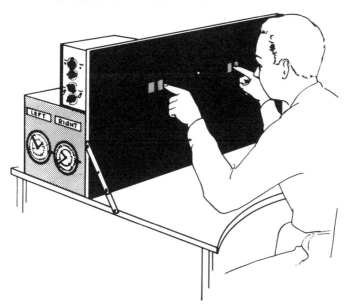

Fig. 11. Apparatus to measure reaction time to visual discrimination presented either singly or simultaneously to each visual field. (From *The Bisected Brain* by M. S. Gazzaniga, 1970. New York: Appleton-Century-Crofts.)

Patients are to some extent able to overcome their difficulties in cross-integration. One patient described by Sperry (1968) was reported to be performing cross-integrational tasks at well above the level of performance during the first year after surgery, and this patient at the time of reporting was continuing to show an improvement.

Also, many of the cross-integrational effects are easily compensated for in everyday behaviour outside the testing situation. Auditory cues, for example, have to be carefully controlled to prevent one hemisphere hearing what the other is doing. The right hand must be kept away from the left hand to prevent the transmission of information by touch, and the patient must be prevented from lifting test objects up to touch the face or the head area. Also, as we shall see later, the patient must be prevented from describing what he is doing in the form of a running commentary, because by these means the left hemisphere can provide the right hemisphere with pertinent information about its functions.

A series of tests were employed (Sperry, 1966, 1968) in which the subject held both hands out of sight with the palm up and the fingers extended. He then pointed with his thumb to spots stimulated by the examiner on different segments of the finger and upper palm. The normal person can generally point to corresponding symmetrical spots on the opposite hand using the opposite thumb. Commissurotomy patients have difficulty in performing this task although some patients appear to be able to carry it out, even after commissurotomy. Also, pictures of finger and thumb postures were flashed on to a screen stimulating one half only of the visual field. Movements of the hand on the same side present no problem but performance is not as easy with the hand on the opposite side, although patients are to some degree able to perform this task. Control of the left hand through the major hemisphere seems to be marginally better than control of the right hand through the minor hemisphere. Each hemisphere can apparently control the movements of both sides including to some extent those of the ipsilateral fingers and hand (Hamilton, 1967).

The first patient on whom the split-brain surgery was performed showed a marked failure of integration across the midline of the body; he could not localize with one hand points touched on the opposite side of the body. In the second case, however, the patient, unlike the first, retained a greater degree of crossed-lateral control. If an object was placed in her left hand whilst she was blindfolded, although she could not name the object she was able to demonstrate its use, and she has the facility to carry out verbal commands with her left hand or her left leg, a function which the previous patient was unable to execute.

Gazzaniga, Bogen and Sperry (1967) describe disturbances of motor function in nine patients, all of whom had undergone surgical disconnection. It is clear from the study of these patients that the capacity for lateral transfer of information in the brain in the absence of the corpus callosum can vary from one individual to another. Gazzaniga, Bogen and Sperry (1967) state that discrepancies in the literature could be accounted for in terms of the different extent to which the ipsilateral motor control mechanisms were disrupted by extra commissural damage. These later patients were able to respond normally with the right hand or foot to stimuli presented in the right visual field, and with the left hand and foot to stimuli presented to the left visual field. When visual input was confined to the same hemisphere as the hand employed to demonstrate the particular task, each hemisphere has a capacity for performance. For example, a spot of light flashed to the right visual field can be pointed to easily with the right hand. Similarly, if a spot of light is flashed to the left visual field then the subject can point to it with his left hand. Both hemispheres are able to identify geometric shapes presented to them by selecting, with the appropriate hand, the correct one amongst a series of alternatives. The left hand in these patients is good at copying geometric forms, suggesting a pre-eminence in the ability to deal effectively with constructional aspects of spatial perception. The right hand proves itself to be inferior at this task, showing selective dyspraxia. Both hands are able adequately to localize stimulus points and to show finely graded mimicking of finger postures from diagrams presented to the appropriate half visual field. Both are able to execute simple commands presented by way of written verbal instructions to the appropriate half visual field, instructions such as 'point, tap, grip', etc.

The earlier observations that the patient was unable to cross-integrate information, and that the right hand had no knowledge of the functions of the left hand, were not entirely confirmed by the results of these subsequent studies. When information was directed to the major hemisphere and response demanded from the subordinate hand, response was usually quite good if it did not demand fine control of finger movements. The patient, for example, could point to an object in the left visual field and could satisfactorily draw its outlines. When printed words were flashed to the left hemisphere they could be written using the left hand. Control, however, tended to break down when fine finger movements were involved. All patients were extremely poor at indicating the matching points on the left side by movements of the thumb and finger of the left hand. Similarly, performance was poor on tests demanding fine finger control on tasks in which the information was directed to the left visual field and response demanded from the right or dominant hand. The results were erratic and failures common. Fairly good results were obtained, however, indicating quite a large degree of transfer even from the right hemisphere to the dominant hand in tasks involving simple gross movements like pointing to an object or tracing the outline of a shape flashed to the left visual field. It is clear that the ideas of total disconnection have not completely withstood this test of subsequent and sustained investigation, although the transport of certain types of information is nevertheless considerably impaired by surgical section.

There is some evidence that left hemisphere functions compete with those of the right. The ipsilateral manual control over the dominant hand by the right hemisphere could easily be disturbed by the influx of fresh information into the left hemisphere, particularly that of contradictory information.

What at first seemed to be a very clear picture of a total failure to integrate information across the midline of the body has had to give place to a less precise although similar account, whereby failure occurs in some patients but in others integration is still possible. Even in these latter patients, however, there is a deterioration in performance. It may be that patients such as those described here with pathological disturbances come to rely on the corpus callosum alone, far more than is normal in order that one hemisphere may be kept in touch with the functions of the other. The term disconnection syndrome in cases such as these is particularly apt as in the first case described by Bogen and Vogel. In other cases it is obvious that the hemispheres are not totally disconnected but transit of some types of information, but not all, is blocked. For example, work in progress but not yet reported in the journals suggests that information about ambient vision, chimeric stimuli and perceptual closure all transfer. The more recent investigations suggest not a total disconnection but a restricted blocking of information transit. Failure to transfer occurs in relation to information for the fine control of motor action, but not that of the coarser grained movements. It appears that the callosum has responsibility for the transfer of complex information. Such a view would conform with the notion that complex functions are performed by the areas most recently elaborated in the history of the evolution of the brain.

PERCEPTUAL PROCESSES

The perceptual processes have been extensively studied in split-brain patients. Stimuli are projected to either the right or the left hemisphere by directing the stimulus material to the right or the left visual field after the subject has fixated a central point.

In experiments previously described a pattern was flashed to either the left or right visual field. The subject was required to point with the right or left hand to the corresponding pattern on a set of five cards placed in front of him. When the stimulus appeared in the left visual field the patient could identify the pattern with his left hand. When the pattern was flashed to the right visual field the patient could identify the stimulus with the right hand or verbally. When stimuli were flashed simultaneously to both fields and each hand responded to its respective stimulus, the percentage of correct retrieval by either hand did not drop (Gazzaniga et al., 1965).

The patients have little appreciable difficulty in analysing the information coming to either the right or the left hemisphere. The difficulty they have arises in relating the information of one hemisphere to that of the other. They are able to transfer information perfectly well from one modality to another within the single hamisphere but they cannot transfer information in the same modality from one hemisphere to the other (Gazzaniga et al., 1965).

Observations of this kind suggest that the mechanisms of perceptual analysis are duplicated within each cerebral hemisphere. The person analyses the information coming from the external world by a complex process, dependent on pre-existing mechanisms and prior experience.

Indeed, if the mechanisms of distance and depth perception are considered, it might be assumed that these involve separate analysis within each cerebral hemisphere of slightly different patterns and to carry out a scrutiny of these it is necessary to have independent analysing systems.

Studies have been undertaken to test speed of hemisphere function in split-brain patients. There is some difficulty in comparing the response times of patients with controls, because patients have brain pathology which may affect their response both before and after section of the callosum. Information about reaction time does not tell us as much as we could hope. Smith (1947) found that reaction times increased after section of the callosum. He was inclined to attribute this to inertia in patients with surgical lesions of the commissural pathways. However, there were no differences in response times to complex visual discriminations or word association tasks and these results would be consistent with the view that the actions within one hemisphere have an arousing effect when transmitted to the other and the lack of continuous feedback is responsible for the effect. More complex stimuli with a higher arousal component compensate for the lack of stimulation from the opposite hemisphere. Against this, however, the fact can be quoted that monkeys with section of the callosum show a greater time in wakefulness than controls (Batini et al., 1966). Smith (1947) studied response times in the crossed and uncrossed condition, i.e. the signal was projected to one hemisphere and the response emanated from the same hemisphere; secondly the response emanated from one hemisphere whereas the signal was projected to the other. There were differences but Smith (1947) does not regard these of a high order. They do suggest, however, that information employs a less direct route in the absence of the callosum and increased response times could be regarded as a measure of this.

In other studies of response time, there is evidence that unlike the normal person, commissurotomy patients carry out double voluntary reaction time tasks as fast as they carry out a single reaction (Gazzaniga and Sperry, 1966). Sperry and Gazzaniga (1966) also studied the extent to which the disconnected hemispheres carry on simultaneous activity by presenting a visual discrimination task to the left hemisphere first and then the same task accompanied by another discrimination task to the right hemisphere. Response times were taken to the single and the double presentation. Lack of interference was characteristic of the double situation. When a red-green discrimination was used in the right visual field and a light-dark discrimination in the left visual field, the double task was performed as rapidly as the single task.

When the cerebral hemispheres have been separated by surgical division, each of the two disconnected hemispheres continues to function much as before, except that a high degree of interdependence between them is no longer possible.

Gazzaniga and Young (1968) found that the split-brain monkey can process and respond to more information involving bimanual motor sequencing than can controls with their commissures intact. Presumably this increase in capacity arises because of the enhanced capacity for independent hemisphere function which did not previously exist. The separation of the hemispheres appears to disconnect the previously cooperating machinery, dividing the brain into two functioning wholes.

Results of this kind point to the hemispheres as two independently functioning mechanisms which nonetheless have links operating between them which normally exert an overriding control. When the links are disrupted each is freed from its responsibility to the other and utilizes the capacity to carry out tasks in its own right. It is possible, as we shall see later that information is preprocessed by each hemisphere and that central integration occurs at a later stage. Experiments of this type point to the capacity, whether latent or not, for each to act as its own analysing system and for each to process independently the information necessary for behavioural control.

Sperry (1968) stated that 'the split-brain animal or person behaves in many ways as if it had two separate brains, each with a mind of its own. In dividing the brain in half the functional properties are not quite divided in the same way. In a very direct sense because of the extensive bilateral duplication, many of the brain functions are doubled rather than they are halved. Many functions get double representation. They are organized on both the right and the left sides. When the hemisphere is released from its reciprocal cross controls, each hemisphere is then free to carry out these respective functions.'

Throughout the literature on hemisphere functions in the human brain, there are reports that different hemispheres are specialized for particular functions. These claims will be examined in more detail in a later chapter; meanwhile our task is to examine the light which studies of section of the corpus callosum throw on this problem. In some of the first observations reported by Bogen and Vogel, it became clear that both of the earlier patients failed to notice stimuli at the left side of the body if at the same time their attention was occupied with a task involving the right hand (Gazzaniga et al., 1963). There seemed to be two possibilities, one that the patient had not noticed the stimulus, or secondly that the patient had noticed the stimulus but failed to respond to it. When it is considered that each hemisphere has some capacity to control each hand, and that after section of the corpus callosum the left hemisphere may retain the capacity to control not only the right, but the left hand as well, it is possible that the left hemisphere by its action blocks the access of the right hemisphere to the left hand and the functions of the right hemisphere can no longer be expressed through that hand. It need not be the case that the hemisphere ceases to attend to the stimuli but rather that its output is blocked.

Gazzaniga and Sperry (1967) suggest that in cases in which the right hemisphere is called upon to perform movements of the right or dominant hand, performance is poor because of competition for right hand control coming from the left. They tested the effect of such competition by presenting a second stimulus to the left hemisphere at the same time as the right hemisphere operated the dominant hand. If contradictory information was presented to the left hemisphere then the right hemisphere was unable to execute its response. Similarly, various shapes could be drawn by the right dominant hand, providing that other shapes were not also at the same time flashed to the left hemisphere. These results seem to confirm the view that response competition operates with regard to the performance of the hands. Gazzaniga and Sperry suggest that the motor output system to the right hand, as might be expected, is in all probability the superior. These results are informative about competing motor output but it should not be assumed that they permit it to be said that the activity of one hemisphere suppresses the capacity of the other to receive information which might be one of the first assumptions.

MEMORY

Evidence from the study of animal behaviour suggests that the memory processes are represented bilaterally. Gazzaniga and Young (1967), as we have already seen, showed that split-brain monkeys are able to remember more of a total situation if some of the information is directed to one hemisphere and the rest directed to the other. Normal monkeys required to push the lit-button of a pair can handle up to six pairs, three in each field after the cue lights have been left on for 600 milliseconds. Split-brain monkeys, however, quickly exceed this limit and showed a capacity to respond to eight pairs of lights left on for only 200 milliseconds. The upper limit achieved by the normal animal is surpassed by the brain bisected animal. A similar condition applies with split-brain patients (Gazzaniga, 1968). The patients did not score particularly well overall, which is not surprising in view of their condition, but whilst stimulation of one hemisphere produces a stable rate of performance, stimulation of both hemispheres results in a near doubling of their scores. The subjects were shown a series of alphabetic letters flashed either to the right or to the left of a central fixation point, and each was required to point to as many of the test letters as could be remembered. These results suggest that the existence of the callosum as an intact system reduces the short-term memory capacity. Gazzaniga (1968) suggests that if the hemispheres are disconnected from each other, then both are freed from the task of keeping the other up to date, and they are therefore free to work to capacity in parallel with each other. Dimond (1969) suggests that there are two mechanisms implicated here: one is the delay which transmission across the corpus callosum produces, the other is the possible queueing of information before inter-hemispheric transmission takes place. Each hemisphere may be involved in inter-hemispheric rivalry which plays a part in the observed relationships. Each hemisphere is receiving information; both could store it and direct a template copy to the other but in doing so it is likely that each hemisphere in dispatching information to the other sets up a rivalry and both find themselves in competition. If this occurs, information held up through delays in transit would be likely to decline.

Gazzaniga quotes the case of the left hemisphere, the speech hemisphere. This has the capacity to describe all the events of the left visual field. It is also possible using this hemisphere when the brain is intact (i.e. the normal callosal brain) to describe the events of the right visual field in addition to those of the left. Information about the right visual field must be transmitted across the corpus callosum in order that it may be described by the left hemisphere. That a duplicate pattern of the visual world of that side is dispatched across is suggested by certain electrophysiological investigations (Gazzaniga et al., 1967; Berlucchi et al., 1967). Investigations of hemispheric refractoriness (Dimond, 1970c) suggest that information is already essentially coded and in an abstract form before its transmission across the callosum.

Milner et al. (1968) report evidence in studies of immediate memory of suppression of input to one hemisphere by the functions of the other. Auditory fibres from each ear are distributed to both hemispheres but with a more pronounced contralateral system. Physiological studies of animals (Tunturi, 1946; Rosenzweig, 1951) have shown that the projection from each ear to the contralateral temporal lobe is greater than to the ipsilateral temporal lobe. Bocca et al. (1955) also demonstrated superiority of the ipsilateral ear in patients with temporal lobe lesions. In spite of this bilateral innervation, it is claimed by Milner et al. in their study, that the left or speaking hemisphere suppresses completely or nearly completely the input from the left ear in commissurotomized patients. The task employed was that described by Broadbent (1958) for the study of immediate memory which presents two streams of digits simultaneously to the subject for subsequent recall. In the experiment described by Milner et al. (1968) different digits were presented simultaneously to the two ears. Normal subjects showed a slight but significant superiority for the use of the right ear. Patients with section of the corpus callosum show an almost complete suppression of the digits presented to the left ear. Under conditions of monaural stimulation, digits from both ears are reported correctly, but those at the left ear are suppressed when accompanied by digits at the right ear.

It seems doubtful, however, that these results tell us much about the respective role of the cerebral hemispheres with regard to the storage of information. It is possible, for example, that the right hemisphere is unable to comment on the information which it receives because, as has been shown, commissurotomized patients are unable to use speech to indicate the functions of the right hemisphere. Milner et al. (1968) required their subjects to state verbally the messages they had received over the headphones. It must be assumed therefore that what is reported are the messages reaching the left hemisphere. This experiment became a more or less direct test of the efficiency of the direct ipsilateral connection of the left ear to the left hemisphere, compared with the contralateral connection of the right ear to that same hemisphere. It is not surprising that the contralateral pathway proved to be the superior in view of the fact that it is commonly regarded as both anatomically and functionally the superior of the two (Kaas et al., 1967).

Audiometric studies were reported on a patient with section of the corpus callosum by Sparks and Geschwind (1968). This patient underwent various dichotic listening tasks and showed 100 per cent extinction of performance on the left ear. Each could, however, perform normally in the monaural condition. Sparks and Geschwind suggest that the callosal pathway is normally the most important for reporting verbal material presented to the left ear in dichotic tasks. In the absence of the callosal pathway the right is unable to express the information it has received through speech, and as many of the dichotic tasks required verbal report, it is expected that there will be no left hemisphere contribution. Once again this experiment presents a more or less direct test of the efficiency of the ipsilateral and contralateral auditory fibres. Ipsilateral from the left ear, and contralateral from the right ear to the right hemisphere. It is again not surprising, in view of what is known about the importance of the contralateral fibres, that these latter should again prove to be the superior.

So far we can assume that right hemisphere functions have not been tested by the method employed by Milner et al. (1968) or by Sparks and Geschwind (1968). It may not be warranted to regard the right ear as belonging exclusively to the left hemisphere, and to suppose that these experiments demonstrate the superiority of the left hemisphere over the right. When in fact the two hemispheres are tested under conditions which might be regarded as competitive, in which both have access to an output channel, right hemisphere functions are not suppressed by auditory input to the left hemisphere. Instruction tapes were prepared which contained not digits but simple commands (Milner *et al.,* 1968). When two messages were presented at the same time, one to each ear, e.g. the right ear might receive the message 'now pick up the paper clip' at the same time that the left ear received the words 'now find us the eraser', then left hand retrieval of objects specified through the left ear with partial to complete neglect of objects named through the right ear was a characteristic feature of performance. This suggests that as regards commands to information, the right hemisphere is at least the equal and has proved itself to be the superior on tasks in which it has an outlet channel through which to express itself. This emphasizes the fact that again the results reported earlier with regard to the suppression of digits presented to the right ear indicate a combination first of the strength of the contralateral pathways and secondly the fact that the right hemisphere was not able to express the information which had been received. The results do not indicate the suppression of right hemisphere functions by those of the left, and where proper provision of a channel is made for the right hemisphere to express its operations, then bearing in mind the relative importance of the contralateral auditory fibres, it may prove itself to be at least the equal if not the superior of the so-called dominant hemisphere.

With regard to the memory processes, it seems likely as Gazzaniga (1968) suggested, that memory processes are located bilaterally, and that those of each side are capable of acting as an independent memory store. Suppression of digits by input to a particular hemisphere may be a false inference arising from a set of rather complicated circumstances.

LEARNING CAPACITY

The capacity to learn is not likely to be greatly affected by section of the corpus callosum. Each hemisphere seems to possess the independent capacity to learn and to store information. In terms of overall capacity to learn, the surgery leaves the patient very much unaffected. The question then arises as to the nature of the transfer of previous learning from one hemisphere to another. Smith (1951) reports the effects upon learning and transfer of learning, of cutting the association pathways of the corpus callosum. Six patients were studied with complete section of the corpus callosum, and two with section of all the commissure except the posterior two-thirds.

Capacity at mirror-drawing and non-visual stylus maze learning was examined. Tasks were learned with the preferred hand and the patients were tested with the other hand afterwards. Transfer was established easily both on maze learning and on mirror-drawing in a fashion which in no way differed from controls. Smith (1951) says that these results support the proposition that 'there is no specific or generalized integrative neural mechanism of the cortex explicitly essential for learning and related functions which nay be rendered seriously inoperative by injury to the particular callosal pathways'.

In the study by Smith (1951) transfer of learned response occurred across the midline, although the corpus callosum had been sectioned. In the light of subsequent studies these results are somewhat anomalous. Several possibilities may be advanced as an explanation. Recovery of the capacity to cross-localize points of stimuli occurs at varying times post-operatively (Sperry, 1968). The brain is able to compensate for the loss of the corpus callosum, and learning to use other pathways is a feature of neural organization. The nervous system may acquire the capacity to re-route information around the brain.

Sperry (1968) advances a number of other reasons as to why information transfer appears on some occasions but not others. The cross-integrational deficits are not all that obvious, and they may be difficult to isolate. Eye-movement scanning can account for some capacity to cross-integrate as well as the use of other sense organs to obtain contralateral information. Movements could be detected across the body by means of both the proprioceptive senses and the body feedback systems. The ears may be used to achieve integration and Sperry, Gazzaniga and others, reported that care must be taken to stop the person talking out loud whilst carrying out an experiment.

SPATIAL FUNCTIONS

It is possible that visuo-spatial functions relate primarily to the right hemisphere. Hughlings Jackson (1874) suggested that 'if it should be proved that the faculty of expression resides in one hemisphere, there is no absurdity in raising the question as to whether perception its corresponding opposite may not be seated in the other'.

When sensory information is projected to the right hemisphere and performance required of the left hand, good performance is achieved on non-verbal tasks. Fine individual finger movement appears. Mimicking of hand, thumb and finger postures is readily demonstrated. Objects like cigarettes, keys, glasses etc., are manipulated correctly with highly refined movements (Sperry, 1968).

The first patient described by Gazzaniga et al. (1963), although never having drawn with his left hand previously prior to the operation, seemed to show greater facility for drawing spatial structures when using his left hand than when using his right. A necker-cube and other spatial patterns were correctly reproduced when the left hand was employed, but the right hand showed very poor performance.

Constructional tasks involving a large spatial component were also performed more proficiently by the left then the right hand. For example, selective dyspraxia of the right hand in carrying out a block

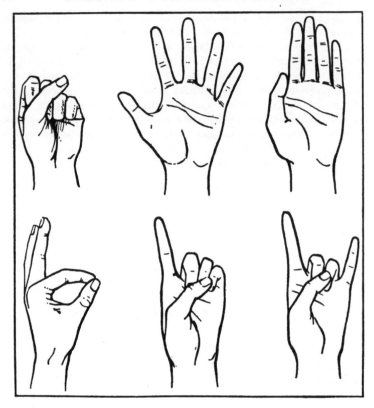

Fig. 12. Sample drawings of different hand positions that were flashed to left or right hemisphere to test ability of each half brain to execute control over ipsilateral or contralateral hand. (From *The Bisected Brain* by M. S. Gazzaniga, 1970. New York: Appleton-Century-Crofts.)

design test not only appeared in the first patient but also to varying degrees in subsequent ones (Gazzaniga *et al.*, 1967). The left hand does consistently well, whereas the right is barely able to do the simplest problems.

The visuo-spatial superiority of the left hand and the verbal inferiority persisted in the first patient for over two years. The second patient, however, reacquired writing in the left hand and drawing in the right hand by the eighth month after the operation (Bogen and Gazzaniga, 1965).

The probability has to be entertained that the right hemisphere has the greater facility for spatial functions. However, it would be unwise to describe the right as the hemisphere which uniquely fulfils the spatial functions for several reasons. Copying diagrams and assembling blocks into patterns may represent only a small part of what are generally regarded as the spatial functions. Much evidence suggests that the right and left hemispheres as well as the sense organs receive disparate information, the analysis of which is used to locate objects in space. There is evidence of the participation of both hemispheres in acting upon spatial information to integrate body movement. It would appear to be misleading to attribute the capacity for analysing the events of the three-dimensional world to one hemisphere only.

LANGUAGE AND SPEECH

The first patient tested by Bogen and Vogel (1962) showed unilateral language lateralization to a marked degree. In the reports of the first cases described by Gazzaniga et al. (1963), when vision was eliminated by the use of a blindfold, the patient was able to localize points of stimulation on the skin. Correct verbal descriptions of points touched were given only for the right side. Verbal descriptions of points touched on the left were inaccurate and appeared to be occasioned by guesswork on the part of the speech hemisphere. Sperry (1968), on the basis of observations of this kind, suggested that the minor hemisphere is in fact mute and is therefore unable to describe verbally the processes which go on within it. It was also the case in a number of other types of observation concerned with temperature discrimination, pain sensitivity and the position sense, that stimulation of the right side of the body could be described in words, whereas that of the left could not. The subject could also name and describe patterns presented to the right visual field, but when questioned about patterns presented to the left visual field he often appeared surprised and claimed that he saw nothing. The patient also was unable to read or describe objects presented to the left half field of vision.

Sperry (1968) states that the impression might be given that the subjects are simply blind or agnostic for the left field of vision, but with further testing it can be shown that these people do indeed identify the left field stimuli, but like a deaf mute they are unable to talk about what they see. Good perception, recognition, comprehension and memory can all be demonstrated in the right if the tasks are arranged such that this hemisphere can express itself in means other than speech, e.g. by manual pointing or other means (Sperry, 1968).

It is clear that the non-language hemisphere has some ability in that when required to point to visual stimuli presented to the left visual field with the left hand, the patient is able to do so. When means other than language are employed this hemisphere is by no means lacking in a command of higher functions. After 24 months the first patient showed greater proficiency in using either hand to locate the visual target in either half field, but he could still not utter verbal descriptions of stimuli in the left visual field. When two stimuli were flashed one to the left and one to the right visual field, he described the stimulus flashed to the right visual field, but at the same time denied any knowledge of the stimulus flashed to the left field. This patient had been interested in reading, but as his condition deteriorated due to the illness, he was forced to give up most reading, except newspaper headlines. After section of the corpus callosum he watched television and read the newspapers. He did, however, complain of difficulty with sustained reading at some 25 weeks after the surgery, largely because the printed words tended to fade from his vision, and to become indistinguishable. When tested it was found that reading was undertaken by the right half field of vision. His right half reading was fairly normal but he was unable to read or describe words or objects by printed name in the left field of vision. The patient was able to distinguish easily using the left hand between such objects as wooden ovals, pyramids and a door latch, whilst wearing a blindfold. He was consistently unable to give a verbal description of such objects unless he held them in the right hand or if the blindfold was removed, in which case he could describe them well, although still holding them in the left hand. This disconnection of language functions has been extensively described by Gazzaniga *et al.* (1963).

A certain degree of caution is necessary in the interpretation of these results. The possibility exists of damage to the hemisphere structure not directly related to corpus callosum section. In this context it has to be remembered that the patient had been ill for a period prior to the operation and that the symptoms associated with brain malfunction had been getting steadily worse.

The second patient showed a very rapid recovery. Not only could this patient after a few weeks point with either hand to touch stimuli on the opposite side of the body, but could state verbally the position of the points where she had been touched on both sides of the body. The persistent severe apraxia to verbal commands observed in the first patient (Gazzaniga *et al.,* 1963) was absent after the first few weeks after the operation. The fact that it was observable during the first few weeks is a point not to be overlooked but the expectancy of a lasting disconnection syndrome was not borne out by this patient. Gazzaniga (1965) states that the most marked difference was seen in the ability of the second case to use either hand in responding to unilateral cerebral input or to verbal instructions.

After examining further cases, the picture has changed a little. Subsequent patients have been able to do some writing with the left hand, and they do have facility to carry out verbal commands with the left hand. With proper testing it is possible to show that these people are neither word blind, word deaf nor tactually alexic as was supposed after the testing of the first patient (Sperry, 1968). For example, if letters or words are flashed on to a screen in the subject's left and right field of vision, and he is asked to describe what he sees, he describes everything in the right half visual field but nothing in the left half visual field. If a word is flashed in the left half field the patient consistently says that he saw nothing on that trial, or just a brief flash of light but some patients, although denying that they have seen anything, may well be able to write the word or act out a command, e.g. nod or smile.

Sperry (1968) suggests that no speech is indicated for the minor hemisphere but the possibility cannot be excluded that the minor hemisphere is capable of triggering at least a few simple words, and perhaps of singing and swearing. Where a few simple words are directed to the minor hemisphere these may well be triggered.

It has long been supposed in the writings on aphasia according to an established viewpoint, that the right deprived of communication with the language mechanisms of the left is both word blind and word deaf. The latter cases suggest that this may not be so. Although the hemisphere may not express comprehension in speech, and to a lesser extent in writing, it does nonetheless show a degree of comprehension of both written and spoken words. For example, the right hemisphere can be employed to choose from a variety of different kitchen objects after hearing that object described as one used for slicing.

The right can also read and understand the meaning of word symbols. Written vocabulary appears to be childlike, but this may be influenced by the difficulty of presenting long stimulus words to the subject. Auditory comprehension is considerably more advanced.

Recovery of language processes following surgery varied widely from one patient to another. Gazzaniga and Sperry (1967) describe the language processes in three patients. They say that in fact 'the first case had sustained considerable brain damage', especially in the right hemisphere, prior to surgery. It was noteworthy also that the language capacity of the right hemisphere in this first case proved to be almost negligible and decidedly inferior to that of other patients. In subsequent cases it was hoped that it would be possible to study cases which reflect more accurately the effects of cerebral disconnection *per se*.

The first case showed a return of elementary speech at about the first month after surgery, and more advanced conversation by about the eighth week. The second patient showed a period of mutism lasting one or two days after surgery. At the third day, however, this patient was talking over the telephone. During the first two weeks after surgery, she displayed a somewhat erratic emotional lability in conversation. The most rapid recovery was seen, however, in a third and younger patient, a right-handed boy aged 12, who had no history of traumatic brain injury. He was a 'bright, affable and generally happy individual with a pre-operative I.Q. of 115 (WISC) scored under anti-convulsant sedation'. This patient was conversing with the hospital staff within 24 hours. He had good comprehension and he was able to recite 'Peter Piper picked a peck of pickled peppers', etc. without any apparent difficulty. By the second day he was feeding himself and was walking around the hospital at the end of the first week. At this time he did display, but only to a small extent, the apraxic difficulty in making voluntary movements with the left hand to verbal commands, but this was only slight and not permanent as in the first case.

These studies show that the right has little, if any, capacity to express itself through speech, but the question of understanding language is a different one from that of the capacity to speak. A person who is mute can understand what is said to him, but is unable to reply. The question arose as to whether the right hemisphere lacked the understanding of language, or whether it lacked the capacity to express through speech the understanding of language that it possessed. It seemed likely, in view of the experiments already described, that the latter was the case. If short words, e.g. cup, pen, orange etc., were flashed tachistoscopically to the left visual field, the subject was able to point with his left hand to the correct object. Similarly, if a picture of a ship was flashed to the left visual field, the subject would pick up a card with 'ship' written on it when using the left hand, although at the same time denying verbally that he had seen anything. It was difficult, of course, by virtue of the limits of the stimulus material, to determine the upper limits of comprehension.

The patients appeared to have a good understanding of the spoken word through the use of the right hemisphere. A test word was spoken by the examiner, and the patient required to press a button when the correct matching noun was flashed to the left visual field. The examiner would also read a phrase, e.g. 'used to tell time' and the patient could select easily the correct word 'clock' out of five words flashed to the left visual field. Patients obviously comprehend the spoken word within the right hemisphere. They are also able to comprehend through tactile input to the right hemisphere language represented in the form of a series of letters for tactual exploration.

When two pictures are projected on to the screen, one in the left half field of vision and the other in the right, e.g. a picture of a pencil on the left and a knife on the right, the subject invariably when asked says that he saw a knife, or if asked to write what he saw, again he writes a knife. However, if the subject reaches out with his left hand to select one object by touch from amongst others, he is capable of selecting the pencil when this picture is flashed to his left visual field (Sperry and Gazzaniga, 1967).

When the subject has retrieved the object correctly with the left hand and is asked what it is, the right hemisphere tends to construct an incorrect answer which frequently has the effect of making the patient wince when the right hemisphere hears the left hemisphere give the wrong answer (Sperry and Gazzaniga, 1967).

A series of ten objects were placed one at a time in the subject's left hand, and a series of thirteen names of objects written on a card were placed in front of the patient. The subjects were able to identify many of the objects correctly by this means. Typically, the subjects would say the name of the object, but if they made a mistake in naming the object as in pointing with the right hand, then the left would jerk up spontaneously to point to the correct answer. Comprehension of spoken words was tested in a similar manner and again the patient showed a command of auditory comprehension.

In other tests a definition was first read aloud by the experimenter after which the subjects explored a series of objects using the left hand without vision, ultimately selecting the correct object. By increasing the complexity of definition it was possible to establish something of the level of comprehension of the minor hemisphere for spoken language although the objects themselves remained fairly simple.

Tests were carried out to observe the facility of the right hemisphere at spelling. The patients were provided with alphabet letters constructed from cardboard. The subject was told a word and then required to spell it using the left hand. Simple familiar words were spelled correctly, but only slowly and with considerable effort, but the level which was achieved at this task tended to be somewhat low.

Sperry (1968) says that such tests 'indicate the presence in this largely unknown, mute, non-communicative minor hemisphere of the cerebral capacity for things like insight, mental association and ideation'. This is largely revealed by the capacity of the right hemisphere not only to select items indicated by a particular instruction, but also to select items that go with a particular stimulus. For example, if a picture of a cigarette is flashed to the right hemisphere and there is no cigarette amongst the group of objects, the subject may choose with the left hand an ashtray or a box of matches selected from among other objects which have no association with the cigarette.

Sperry (1968), whilst stating that 'no speech is indicated for the minor hemisphere', at the same time suggests that the possibility cannot be excluded that in tests where a choice of only two of three simple words is involved and these have been spoken and prompted by the examiner, there are strong indications in some studies that the minor hemisphere can then trigger speech for the correct word.

The evidence points to the view that the right hemisphere in its linguistic capacity is by no means a word blind, word deaf member. Results suggest that both hemispheres have the capacity to receive information with regard to language functions from the outside world. They have the capacity to analyse that information and to integrate it into nervous system processes which can be expressed although not always through the speech system.

CALCULATION

Sperry (1968) suggested at one time that the ability to calculate appeared to be almost totally missing from the right hemisphere. It appeared, for example, that in non-verbal tests the minor hemisphere was unable to do a simple subtraction task, taking two numbers from under ten. However, in some of the early patients the possibility of damage to the right hemisphere prior to surgery cannot be ruled out, and it may be that to this can be attributed the deficit in calculation. In more recent work Sperry and Biersner (reported by Sperry, 1968), using different testing procedures, moderately good addition, subtraction and multiplication for at least small numbers under twenty have been obtained. Levy-Agresti (1968) also reports evidence for the ability to calculate in the right hemisphere. The subjects were required to indicate the answer using their left hand to sums involving the product of numerals projected to the left visual field. Once again, the output factor appears to be an important one in limiting the expression of what the right hemisphere can perform.

DIFFERENTIAL PERCEPTUAL CAPACITIES

The two hemispheres may function by the employment of quite different modes of response, and it may be that each uses a different strategy in dealing with the events of the world. Evidence about strategies tends to be inferential and it cannot always be affirmed that differential successes are the result of the application of different strategies. However, Levy-Agresti and Sperry (1968) suggest on the basis of their studies of problem solving, that different strategies are in fact employed by the hemispheres.

Thirteen sets of wooden blocks were constructed, three blocks in each set. The blocks resembled one another, but differed according to one salient feature, e.g. how many sides were rough or smooth, relationships of grooves and holes, etc. Thirteen cards were prepared which showed the three blocks in the set. The subject task was to feel one block, using either his right or left hand, and specify which one of the three shown on the card he had been given. Of five commissurotomized patients, three failed on a preliminary investigation. Levy-Agresti and Sperry specify right hemisphere neurological damage as the cause of this failure.

In the other patients there was no neurological or behavioural evidence of hemisphere damage. The left hand was correct on 52 per cent of the trials, the right hand on 20 per cent. Although two patients represent an extremely small sample, and although each patient received only 39 trials, it did appear from this rather limited evidence that the items on which the patient failed were not the same in the case of the right and the left hand. The performance of the right hemisphere from the patterns of successes and failures resembled more closely that of another person than its partner the left. The right showed itself to have proficiency on those sets which had complex qualities and which could readily be visualized, whereas the left succeeded on block sets which needed careful analysis, failing on those which demanded a more immediate grasp of spatial relationships.

This led to the suggestion (Levy-Agresti and Sperry, 1968) that the hemispheres adopt different strategies. The right with its grasp of spatial relationships apprehends events in a Gestalt fashion, whereas the left carries out a sequential analytic procedure. The capacity to apprehend in Gestalt terms raises questions about the supposed functional inferiority of the right. Can it be that a hemisphere acting in this capacity is at the same time manifestly inferior in performance to its companion the left? Even if the capacity to abstract the stimulus Gestalt as Levy (1969) describes it can be explained as nothing more than a difference in the speed of functioning, it is nonetheless significant that the most immediate response should come from the right.

Levy (1969) supposes that language during the course of evolution became involved in antagonism with the processes of perception. This is a questionable point of view because much spatial perception is concerned with the analysis of sequences of events in space as is much language perception. However, in support of the argument, Levy (1969) quotes an experiment which shows that in left-handed people having speech partially represented in both hemispheres (at least supposedly) performance I.Q. showed a considerable decrement. It was argued that the invasion of language processes interferes with the perceptual abilities involved in Gestalt apprehension.

It is possible that left-handers, showing as they do a greater incidence of true mixed-handers among their ranks, to some extent lack the sophisticated specialization for motor output which occurs in a person of more decided lateral preference. It is commonly supposed that inadequate lateralization leads to clumsiness and disturbance in performance of spatial tasks. It may be that the failure of left-handers to perform well on tasks of spatial function could also be attributed to this source.

CONSCIOUSNESS

We have seen plenty of evidence that higher mental processes are to be found both in the left and in the right hemisphere. Sperry (1965) reviewed the evidence on the cases studied to that date and as a natural extension of his system of viewing the functions of the split brain as equivalent to two persons within the same body he made the natural transition to describe the split-brain person as possessing two separate spheres of consciousness. He supposed that all the evidence from the fields of perception, cognition, volition, learning and memory, suggested that the surgery has left these people with two separate minds, i.e. two spheres of consciousness.

Sperry (1968) suggests that each hemisphere not only has its own sphere of consciousness, but it also has a will of its own which directs the function of its hand. On occasions the intentions of the left and the right come into conflict. Sperry, in quoting the first case, states that the patient when dressing, whilst pulling on his trousers with one hand, may find his other hand is at the same time attempting to take them off, or that one hand having just tied the cord on his dressing gown has its efforts frustrated by the other hand which now unties the knot. Instances of this kind are reported, but generally there were so many factors unifying the responses of the two hands that they were comparatively rare.

Sperry (1966) points out that there is a very real division between the experienced contents of the right and the left hemisphere. Whilst many factors ensure unity of experience, for example occupation of the same body ensures that much experience is similar in form, nonetheless, after disconnection it is perfectly possible for each hemisphere to store totally different types of experience and for each to remain unaware of the mental world of the other. Sperry (1968) on the basis of the storage of different types of experience, regards the syndrome as showing an apparent doubling in most of the realms of conscious awareness. 'Each hemisphere appears to have its own separate and private sensations, its own concepts, and its own impulses to act. The evidence suggests that consciousness runs in parallel in both the hemispheres of the split-brain person' (Sperry, 1966).

It has previously been suggested that one hemisphere, the right, behaves mainly as an automaton, a true and unified consciousness being preserved only on the dominant side (Eccles, 1965). Sperry (1968) finds himself in disagreement with this view, and supports the idea that the right has every claim to consciousness as has the left. Sperry (1968), for example, quotes an experiment which illustrates emotional responses on the part of the right. When the patient was performing a visual recognition task a pin-up shot of a nude was flashed to the right. The right responded by causing the patient to blush and to giggle, an 'inner grin' spreading over his face. Also, when the right knows a correct answer and it hears the left in the absence of correct knowledge make a stupid verbal mistake which the left cannot possibly know is a mistake, it triggers a look of pained annoyance across the features. Thus, in all of these cases there is definite evidence that one hemisphere may work out of phase with another, and that distinct differences may be observed in the emotional expressions of the hemispheres at any one time. Whether this signifies a different realm of consciousness is difficult to say. Perhaps Sperry, in talking of a sphere of consciousness, is using the term in the sense of a 'thing' and perhaps it is best retained for a process. Sperry could argue that the process is different, and he could quote his own work in support of such a view. Certainly he has shown that there are differences of a profound type in content as manifested by the left and the right. Whether these can be described as differences in consciousness will still remain inevitably a matter for debate.

CONCLUSIONS

Whilst it appears true that each hemisphere possesses its own perceptual learning and memory mechanisms, the information available in one hemisphere may not be available to the other. In both the animal and the human brain, disconnection of the hemisphere has marked effects on the capacity to cross-integrate information. This is also true in cases of agenesis of the corpus callosum.

Patients are able to point with the right hand to a stimulus source on the right side of the body, but are unable to point the same hand to a source on the left side. When stimuli are projected to one hemisphere alone, either the right or the left, the opposite hemisphere shows itself incapable of responding to those stimuli. The commissurotomy patient can carry out a double voluntary reaction time task as fast as the normal individual can carry out a single response. In tests of memory, stimulation of both hemispheres results in a near doubling of scores. Speech appears to be carried out by the left hemisphere, and visuo-spatial functions in large measure by the right. The patient can describe in speech, information presented to the left hemisphere but not that projected to the right. At the same time the right hemisphere shows linguistic capacities if these are tested by other means.

We have witnessed a reappraisal of the functional significance of the corpus callosum since the early days when it seemed, from the work of Akelaitis and his co-workers, that it had little importance. It is now widely accepted that it does play a major part in the integration of information from both sides of the brain. However, the remarkable coordination of body movements in the everyday behaviour of patients with section of the corpus callosum suggests that some integration of function between the hemispheres is still possible, even in the absence of this structure. Compensatory processes occur over time after surgery. One hemisphere becomes skilled at gathering information about the functions of the other. Also, the possibility exists that mid-brain transit pathways come to take over more and more of the functions formerly subsumed by the callosum.

On the grounds that highly coordinated body movement may be achieved immediately after section of the callosum, and in view of the evidence that compensatory processes come to bear, we may not be wholly justified in the assumption that one hemisphere is totally devoid of contact with the other. It is perhaps more circumspect to regard section of the corpus callosum as a breakdown of communications rather than as total divorce, so that while transit of information concerned with low-level skills or transit of information for emergency reactions may be possible, transmission for highly abstracted tasks is excluded.

Even so, it is still justifiable to talk of disconnection in this sense and the term 'disconnection syndrome' has been employed (Geschwind, 1965). There are behavioural symptoms associated with the syndrome which make the term fully justified.

5

Hemispherectomy

INTRODUCTION

Hemispherectomy is the surgical procedure by which one cerebral hemisphere is removed. It is a source of valuable information about the functions of the cerebral hemispheres and is carried out on animals to study experimentally the control which the remaining hemisphere exercises over behaviour. It is also used for the removal of tumour in human beings and for treatment of intractable epilepsy particularly in association with infantile hemiplegia. By studying such cases it is possible to gather information about the tandem arrangement of the brain, and about the functions of one hemisphere in the absence of the other.

EFFECTS OF HEMISPHERECTOMY AND UNILATERAL CEREBRAL LESIONS IN ANIMALS

The first point to be noted about this form of surgery in animals is that it induces a variety of motor disturbances (Popov, 1953; Kellogg, 1948). Hemi-decorticate dogs show a persisting rigidity of the limbs on the opposite side to that of the lesion. This entails some disturbance of reflex patterns and is frequently accompanied by bizarre and seemingly awkward postures. These are not permanent and Kellogg (1949) argues that it is necessary to allow time following unicortical ablation to observe the restructuring of the brain's influence over locomotor abilities.

Cats also have been studied in the hemi-decorticate condition. Their hopping and placing reactions are controlled by cortical areas on the contralateral side to the limbs involved in the response (Bard, 1933). It was thought at one time that these responses could not occur in the absence of the appropriate area of the cortex. However, after removal of the forebrain on one side, the placing response may disappear temporarily but after a short period it returns (Bogen and Campbell, 1960) and recovery takes place even after total hemispherectomy (Bogen and Campbell, 1962). After unilateral forebrain removal the possibility exists that the hindbrain may establish control. In hemispherectomy this is ruled out, because of the absence of both the forebrain and the hindbrain on the one side. This shows that motor control can be maintained although the normal system is no longer functional. The one hemisphere extends the mantle of its control after damage to the other and each can substitute through the use of ipsilateral fibres for many functions of the other. Each has potential to exercise control over the motor responses of the whole organism and following hemispherectomy much of this is realized. The development of control by the ipsilateral hemisphere is not as surprising as it may at first seem because of the presence of the uncrossed fibres.

The question arises as to whether substitution can occur for learned motor response. As is well known, either the right or the left limb can be conditioned to respond to appropriate stimuli but if conditioned responses are laid down before complete hemispherectomy they are disturbed following surgery (Serkov et al., 1966). About one month later they return in full force to the pre-operative level. The disturbance of motor function is transitory. Presumably subsequent improvement reflects the capacity of the single remaining hemisphere to exercise control of both lateral regions.

The perceptual deficits are equal and opposite across the hemispheres. They not only accompany but in some cases are responsible for other types of deficiency. For example, Kellogg (1949) showed that dogs fail to walk in a straight line and circle towards the side of the lesion following removal of one occipital lobe. Circling movements disappear after an interval of three to four months. After this interval the animal walks in a straight line but with some impairment because of the continued absence of reflex patterns. The circling movements cease with recovery of motor control and the resumption of visual function.

The effect of hemispherectomy on position response bias was studied by Kruper et al. (1965). Monkeys were required to discriminate between two wooden blocks of different thickness, between squares of different brightness, or to recover food rewards attached to one of four pieces of string indicated by a patterned area. Surgical removal of the right hemisphere was accompanied by a right position ,bias, and discriminations were somewhat less effective. There are several factors to be considered; first, a position bias will act as a disruptive factor and secondly the animal may suffer initial perceptual disturbances. Also both hemispheres may normally cooperate together in discrimination to enhance performance. In the absence of one this may no longer be possible and the function is performed at an inferior level.

There are also changes in eye function following hemispherectomy. After removal of either the right or the left hemisphere monkeys show a preference for the use of the eye on the same side as that of the removed hemisphere, in spite of the fact that both eyes project fibres to the remaining hemisphere (Kruper *et al.,* 1967). This suggests a preference for the temporal retina with its direct connection to the intact hemisphere rather than the nasal of the other eye with its lateral crossed connection. It is worth noting that cerebral lesions may result in unexpected changes, for example the eyes follow a stimulus smoothly when it moves towards a field defect but irregularly when it moves away from the defect, because of damage to oculomotor centres in the parietal region.

Visual discriminations and eye preference are not the only capacities to be affected. Lobanova (1966) studied the effects on spatial localization. Dogs were trained using conditioned motor-alimentary responses to respond to sounds at frequencies of 500 c.p.s. (spatially distributed) at two food boxes to the right and to the left and also to a metronome at a food box in the middle. Previously established responses were disturbed after hemispherectomy and the animal showed profound spatial disorientation. After a period of 3—5 weeks correct responses began to appear once again and to all outward appearances at that time the function of spatial analysis had been restored. The intact hemisphere apparently compensates for the loss of the other and the single hemisphere appears to exercise the functions which formerly would have employed the two.

Many motor and perceptual functions which normally are controlled by both hemispheres can, under these circumstances, be carried out by one. Some potential for function remains and this suggests that the nervous control is not completely fixed or rigid even in the adult animal.

Plasticity of neural function may relate to the capacity to learn. Investigations are reported of learning in hemi-decorticate animals. Bilateral extirpation prevents the establishment of fresh conditioned responses and eliminates previously established ones. This is not so in the unilateral case and following ablation of the contralateral motor cortex the leg opposite to that previously conditioned to respond now flexes to a tone although shock is still applied to the original limb (Shurrager, 1941). This substitute response occurred shortly after surgery moreover and a long recovery period was unnecessary. In the investigations of Whatmore and Kleitman (1946) it was also shown that hemi-decortication may not only abolish a conditioned response in one limb but frequently the animal lifted the opposite limb instead.

Pribram *et al.* (1964) found that after training a dog to raise its right hind leg to a particular signal the application of strychnine sulphate to the dominant neural focus for the left foreleg resulted in the lifting not of the right foreleg, the response to which the animal had been trained, but the left foreleg. This shows that it is possible to switch motor output from one side of the body to the other. This suggests that there are replicated centres of motor control within each hemisphere and that one can function in place of the other should the occasion demand.

Following unilateral cortical ablation it commonly happens that one limb is used in preference to the other. Cats required to draw food towards themselves with one forelimb, showed a preference for the use of the ipsilateral limb after unilateral ablation of the sensori-motor cortex (Jankowska and Gorska, 1960). That is not to say that the other forelimb could not be employed. When food reward was withheld from the ipsilateral limb, the other limb came into its own and was used proficiently to obtain the food. The use of one limb may be overshadowed by the use of the other, but after unilateral ablation the former may still be used should the need arise.

The resumption of control by the remaining hemisphere of functions which must be presumed to have been formerly exercised by the other, is strong evidence for duplication of function in the animal brain. Each hemisphere may not only assume control over previously learned tasks, but may also accommodate new learning. Each one may act as effectively as the other, but can one hemisphere act as effectively as two? Oakley and Russell (1968) found that the acquisition of the conditioned nictating membrane response did not differ significantly in hemi-decorticate animals from those with both hemispheres intact. This can be interpreted in line with previous work that each hemisphere in the animal brain has considerable potential for fresh learning, and that no one hemisphere has the monopoly.

Studies of electrical activity have been used to determine the influence of one hemisphere on the functional state of the other. Removal of one initially alters the cortical activity of the other (Serkov and Makul'kin, 1965). Fast small potentials are reduced and there is a marked increase of large slow potentials (7-12 c.p.s.) together with characteristic spindle bursts. These changes are not permanent and after four or five days activity tends to return to normal. Slow activity is reduced and fast small potentials increase once again. The development of some electrical changes characteristic of sleep may suggest that each hemisphere in the normal brain has an activating effect upon the other through their joint action on subcortical structures. Many of the initial changes, e.g. the abolition of desynchronization (activating influences) may be due to this lack of activation. Subsequent recovery in the state of electrical activity represents a functional reorganization in response to this.

Studies of hemispherectomy in animals support the view of the brain as a duplicate system. Removal of one hemisphere, whilst not leaving the animal totally unaffected, does not have the serious consequences that might at first be supposed. Each hemisphere is capable of assuming many functions of the other, and indeed, after a time, the organism may begin to approach normal levels of function. There is no substantial evidence of asymmetry in brain function and little evidence that one hemisphere directs the functions of the other. The arrangement appears to be a true partnership, but one with duplication of function and potential for unitary function should the occasion demand.

HEMISPHERECTOMY IN MAN

The term hemispherectomy applied to man may be a misnomer in that strictly speaking the whole of the hemisphere is not removed. In reality decortication occurs. The frontal, parietal, occipital, and temporal lobes except for the small portion lying on the medial surface are removed. Part of the thalamus and part of the basal ganglia may remain.

Hemispherectomy is undertaken for two major conditions. The first of these is tumour which invades most of the hemisphere. Dandy (1928, 1933) introduced hemispherectomy for the treatment of this condition.

It is also employed in the treatment of infantile hemiplegia. Carmichael (1966) lists the indications as follows: 'The patient must first of all have a hemiplegia. This should affect the arm more profoundly than the leg, and the patient usually suffers from fits which do not prove amenable to medical treatment. The patient frequently has behaviour disturbances in the nature of being difficult to handle, personality problems, temper tantrums and rages.'

It is important to differentiate between the infantile hemiplegia and the glioma cases. In the former the hemisphere is removed to treat a condition arising early in the life of the individual. Here there is evidence for considerable duplication of potential for function. When damage occurs to one hemisphere at an early age the other is capable of making considerable restitution. When on the other hand the brain of the adult is rapidly invaded by pathological tissue as happens in glioma, there is far less potential for relearning and restitution and the clinical picture is a different one.

Systematic evidence may be difficult to collect from cases of this kind. The indications for hemispherectomy are gross pathology, either hemiplegia, tumour or focal epilepsy and subsequent behaviour may not be free from the effects which this originally exerted. The fact remains that evidence however equivocal is available from this source and our task is to review this in more detail.

ELECTRICAL ACTIVITY

Obrador and Larramendi (1950) carried out observations on electrical rhythms after surgical removal of a cerebral hemisphere. They quote the evidence obtained from a patient, an 18-year-old girl with a right sided hemispherectomy. This was followed immediately by the cessation of seizures for which she was being treated. After a while the E.E.G. from the remaining left side approached normality, at the same time the E.E.G. from the operated side indicated the presence of physically conducted electrical rhythm. The E.E.G. also revealed a stimulation effect from this half of the brain indicating some ipsilateral projection to the sensory cortex. This patient had tactile sensations on her left side and could indicate when stimulation was taking place. Marshall and Walker (1950) also report evidence of E.E.G. function following right hemispherectomy in four patients. In all cases a rhythm in the range of alpha activity was present on the hemispherectomized side, but in three cases the voltage of the activity was reduced on that side. Weiss et al. (1956) report in the case of a patient showing the loss of the right hemisphere due to natural causes that stimuli could be recognized emanating from the left side of the body and that in this particular patient unremitting pain was experienced from this region.

In the ten cases reported by Obrador (1964) the post-operative E.E.G. was normal in six cases showing only slight changes subsequent to hyperventilation. In the other four patients the E.E.G. showed persistent anomalies including theta rhythms with spikes and discharges, theta activity with large spikes, or records with large voltage delta waves and atypical complexes of spike and slow wave.

Nocturnal E.E.G. patterns have been studied in patients following complete or partial hemispherectomy (Mingrino et al., 1969). Complete hemispherectomy for infantile spastic hemiplagia with epilepsy was carried out on four patients and partial hemispherectomy on three patients. Partial hemispherectomy did not induce significant alterations of E.E.G. patterns during nocturnal sleep, but the tracings of patients with complete hemispherectomy were characterized by the absence of phase IV sleep and a reduced percentage and late appearance of rapid eye movement sleep.

It might be supposed that removal of one hemisphere could result in permanent disruption of the functions of the other, and in electrical silence over the site of removal. This was not the case. Subcortical regions may to some extent be implicated, but the appearance of a record from the absent brain can be attributed to simple conduction in the cortico-spinal fluid which fills the hemicranium (McFie, 1961). The fact that the disruption of electrical activity in the preserved hemisphere occurred as a temporary manifestation in most cases suggests that each hemisphere following the loss of the other readjusts its function to accord with the fresh demands placed upon it.

MOTOR BEHAVIOUR

Some patients who received injury to one hemisphere at or around the time of birth show hemiplegia accompanied by epilepsy which in some cases is severe. If one hemisphere was damaged when the person was young, as regards the symptoms it makes little difference whether this be the right or the left except of course that the lateral position of the hemiplegia will vary. Trauma leading to hemiparesis in most cases occurs early in life many years previous to the hemispherectomy. It might be expected that the removal of one cerebral hemisphere would have profound effects upon motor behaviour. In fact in these cases it appears to leave the patients' motor behaviour unaffected over the longer term (Dandy, 1933; Krynauw, 1950a, b; Mackay, 1952).

In the series of infantile hemiplegia cases studied by French and Johnson (1955a) all had become hemiparetic many years previously. Shortly after recovery from the anaesthetic most could make movements of a gross kind with the previously unaffected arm and leg. The previously spastic limbs were completely flaccid, but reflexes and toe signs were still hyperactive. Within one week two patients were walking unassisted and the other six did so within two to four weeks post-operatively. The average time required to regain walking ability was twelve days.

In the beginning of the series only severe cases were chosen; in the latter part less severe cases were studied. The degree of additional post-operative hemiparesis was, in fact, minimal. Removal of the entire cerebral cortex as well as most of the basal ganglia did not result in exaggeration of the previous motor defect. It was believed that the rapid return of motor function to the pre-operative level was due to the contralateral hemisphere having assumed the function of the pathological side many years pre-operatively (French and Johnson, 1955b).

Ability to use the affected arm also returned to the pre-operative level, but somewhat more slowly than leg function. Finger movement was not abolished by hemispherectomy and all patients were able to move each of their fingers voluntarily. The fingers, however, could be moved with greater facility than the thumb. Post-operatively one patient remarked that he could use his hand and arm without purposely thinking about it as was necessary before.

The immediate post-operative state of the affected side was at first one of complete flaccidity although the reflexes remained hyperactive.

As motor activity returned, the affected side became more spastic and in a period varying from one to nine months the spasticity was comparable to the previous level.

It is clear from this work that patients who develop cerebral pathology in one hemisphere early in life are not greatly affected when the hemisphere which is the origin of the malfunction is removed. Obrador (1964) quoted evidence to show not only that there are no signs of further disturbance in limbs which were not previously affected by the hemiplegia but also that the activities of the formerly hemiplegic side remain virtually unchanged. There may be some indication of a slight increase in muscle tone and some increase of the activity of the typical pyramidal reflexes, but that is essentially all.

The ineffective hemisphere may no longer have a deleterious influence on behaviour. The capacities which were formerly invested with it are likely to have been transferred to the other side many years previously.

It is possible that walking as a pattern of movement is laid down largely in the spinal cord. Sherrington showed that walking and standing are possible in the spinal animal. Travis and Woolsey (1956) also showed that if proper care is provided then a monkey will right itself and walk although the neocortex is removed. Whilst much automatic movement could be patterned by the spinal cord the responsibility for the initiation and control of walking may well be vested at a higher level. As regards hemiplegic patients it appears that control of walking may be exercised and possibly has been for many years by the intact hemisphere.

Movements of the eyes, the tongue, the neck and the trunk remain unaffected by hemisphere removal, whether it be the right or the left. Control, it seems now, rests exclusively with the effective hemisphere. Each providing it remains undamaged is capable of this. Obrador (1964) quotes evidence from cases of both right and left hemispherectomy. Some patients show slight facial paresis observed usually in emotional circumstances, and in others there was a moderate lower facial paresis but in all cases this was minimal.

The remarkable facility of the single hemisphere in innervating the facial muscles was demonstrated by the fact that four patients had the capacity to move selectively any of the contralateral facial muscles. This illustrates the capacity of the hemisphere to exert finely graded and differentiated control over contralateral and ipsilateral motor systems.

Obrador (1964) comments that the motor pattern after the removal of an atrophic cerebral hemisphere shows both positive and negative features. Innervation of the distal parts of the limbs (hand and foot) may be rather poor but the residual mobility which allows the individual to walk and to perform differentiated facial movements is noteworthy and each hemisphere shows the ability in the control of these functions. Bates (1953) produced both contralateral and ipsilateral movements by electrical stimulation in the prerolandic region of the remaining hemisphere immediately after hemispherectomy. It is not clear, however, if this is the normal state of affairs or whether it mirrors the migration of function away from a diseased to a healthy hemisphere. The evidence suggests that most movement patterns apart from the highly discriminative ones of the extremities can be controlled by the single remaining hemisphere. As has been pointed out the subcortical patterning of movements contributes to this process, nonetheless, in many respects one hemisphere is effective as a motor organizer for both the ipsilateral and contralateral sides of the body, and the fact that this is true whether it be the left or right suggests a large equivalence of potential in the developing brain.

The cases of infantile hemiplegia suggest that until a certain age either hemisphere may become invested with the functions of the other should the latter become diseased. Beyond that age, however, the potential for transfer becomes reduced, and studies of pathology in the adult throw light on the changes of plasticity in brain structure which come about with age.

Where hemispherectomy is used in the adult for the treatment of tumour having a rapid history of onset the motor functions are less plastic and when the motor cortex is destroyed on one side a lasting hemiplegia may occur on the other. In such patients there is little useful function in the arm, although the leg may not be as severely affected (Weiss et al., 1956). Obrador (1964) states, however, that in cases of glioma no serious difficulties are reported in walking following hemispherectomy. This suggests that the capacity of one hemisphere to take over or relearn the functions of the other has become reduced with age. The presence of hemiparesis is convincing evidence of double representation of motor functions but the older patient appears to have lost much of the ability to relearn new patterns of control.

PERCEPTION

There are obvious defects in some processes of perception following hemispherectomy but in general the effect upon the sensory systems and the capacity to perceive is limited because of extensive bilateral duplication.

The effect upon hearing in infantile hemiplegia patients has been studied by a number of authors. Goldstein et al. (1956) report in a study of four patients on whom left hemispherectomies had been performed, that the capacity to discriminate pure tones remained unchanged. Goldstein (1961) carried out a follow-up study of one of the patients. Hearing levels were still normal in both ears for pure tones. There was, however, some deterioration of hearing for high tones, but Goldstein was inclined to attribute this to an unassociated deficit, although Hodgson (1967) also reports the case of a 17-year-old girl who, whilst showing hearing sensitivity for pure tones which was within normal limits bilaterally, also showed a small reduction in sensitivity to high frequencies which was greater in the left ear. It may be that both hemispheres are necessary to the perception of high frequency tones, but no obvious effect is to be observed upon the capacity to hear pure tones of lower frequency.

In view of the association of speech with one hemisphere, it is interesting to note that after hemispherectomy the perception of ordinary speech remains virtually unaffected in infantile hemiplegic patients irrespective of which hemisphere has been removed. Presumably the perception of speech as well as the capacity to speak has been acquired by the remaining hemisphere consequent upon early brain damage. There is normal hearing for unmasked speech (Goldstein et al., 1956; Goetzinger and Angell, 1965) and patients can recognize speech adequately, but they may show a deterioration if the speech is distorted, or occurs against a background of noise. Hodgson (1967) states that discrimination of loud speech was good, but with distorted speech, discrimination in both ears was lower than the expected norm. Patients tend to perform relatively poorer on the ear contralateral to the lesion with filtered or distorted speech. These findings support the view that the contralateral pathways are the most important. They also show that in infantile hemiplegia cases one hemisphere is sufficient for the recognition of speech, either the right or the left, but when demands are made beyond those of the normal as in speech filtering, then deterioration takes place. This suggests that both hemispheres in the normal double brain may be implicated in separating out the auditory message from noise and distortion. Presumably the extra volume of brain tissue of another hemisphere permits a finer analysis than would otherwise be possible.

There is some evidence from audiological analysis that loudness adjustments are disturbed. In matching tones a patient studied by Hodgson (1967) was found to show derecruitment, i.e. although the threshold of the two ears was identical, a tone of only 35 dB was required in the left ear to equal the loudness of the 60 dB in the right ear. On the other hand, adjustment of loudness to produce a mid-plane sensation appears to be relatively unaffected by hemispherectomy. Loudness may be evaluated at a high level within the nervous system, and localization at a lower level. This view has a lot to commend it and if correct, the disturbance of the interaural loudness relationship in the presence of normal localization could be used to suggest higher cortical disturbance. It is also possible that by virtue of its importance to spatial orientation, localization is a function which is rapidly transferred from a diseased hemisphere to a healthy one, and a function furthermore which is accomplished thereafter by the single hemisphere. In spite of the deterioration of loudness evaluation, it is still the case that near normal auditory function persists after extensive damage to ,one hemisphere.

The extent to which one hemisphere can accomplish other functions formerly subsumed by the two has been studied by Obrador (1964) who reports that drawings of simple structures were performed without any obvious sensory disturbance. There were no definite alterations of the body schema, agnosias, apraxias or other disturbance of higher-level sensory motor integration and appropriate visual discriminations were made easily on a conditioning task in which shock to the hand was paired with visual signals (lights of different colours). Discrimination between the different colours was made without difficulty, and conditioning was rapidly established. Some attempts were made to test visual acuity but this again showed no obvious deterioration. Hemianopia is produced by hemispherectomy, however. This is brought about if the patients were not hemianopic before, and may well give rise to disturbances of reading (Carmichael, 1966).

There are a number of reports on tactual and sensory perception in the arm and the leg (French et al., 1955; Gardner et al., 1955; Krynauw, 1950). These emphasize that the amount of sensation retained varies according to how much sensation was lost before surgery. An individual who previously had a definite reduction in sensory perception for a period of time seems to have less deficit following hemispherectomy. One explanation advanced of this is that most of the sensory apparatus for perception relative to the limbs has been assumed by the undamaged hemisphere. As the pathology moves in, so the functions are transferred or relearned. With regard to the other senses, all the patients tested by Obrador (1964) retained their perception of tactile, thermal and painful stimuli applied to the skin, contralateral to the hemispherectomy, although apparently the stimuli were perceived with less intensity than those on the other side. The facial area showed virtually no loss of sensitivity and there were no marked differences between one side of the face and ,the other. Localization of stimuli was good in nearly all the patients, as was the discrimination of figures and symbols drawn upon the skin.

Two point skin threshold gave higher values on the affected side; and whilst the ability to perceive vibratory stimuli was present in some cases, its sensitivity was reduced on the side contralateral to the excision. Position sense was still present, although mistakes were often made on the affected side. Sensory perception generally was disturbed more on the contralateral arm than on the face or the leg. The perception of pain stimuli appears to be preserved on both sides of the body (Weiss *et al.,* 1956). The fibres subserving noxious stimuli are extremely diffuse in the brain stem, and there seems little reason why such fibres should not terminate ipsilaterally in a patient whose contralateral cortex has been gradually deteriorating.

In summary the first point worthy of note is that the patient is able to continue with almost all of those activities which were performed formerly and which depend on the integrity of the sensory and perceptual systems. The second point concerns the fact that the existing hemisphere is capable of taking over the monitoring and control of the perceptual processes which ordinarily would be present in the hemisphere now removed.

LANGUAGE AND SPEECH

Great interest has been expressed in the way in which brain organization relates to language and speech functions. One of the greatest contrasts in the study of hemispherectomy is that between patients treated for epilepsy with infantile hemiplegia, and those treated for adult glioma. The difference lies not in the perceptual and sensory functions but in the field of language and speech. When damage occurs to a hemisphere early in life whether it be the right or the left, there is usually little language loss following hemispherectomy, presumably because functions have been displaced from a deteriorating hemisphere or relearned by the remaining intact one. Transfer or relearning of speech appears to be the rule rather than the exception until the stage of adolescence. Functional plasticity is still marked and stereotyping and fixity of brain organization is not yet a limiting factor. Furthermore, speech is acquired whether the early damage occurs to the right or to the left hemisphere.

In the follow-up study by Goldstein (1961) of a patient with infantile hemiplegia, on whom a left hemispherectomy had been performed, a recording of the patient's speech had been made at the time of the first post-operative test five years previously and was available for comparison with his current speech. His understanding of conversation and his own expressive speech had obviously not deteriorated. His articulation was normal, he was not aphasic, and his vocabulary and language were commensurate with his level of education. There are several cases of infantile hemiplegia in which it is reported that speech three or more years after hemispherectomy was at least as good or better than it was pre-operatively (Falconer, 1960; Feld, 1957; Rosier and Choppy, 1956). Carmichael (1966) reports that of a group of 44 infantile hemiplegia patients all had learned to speak perfectly well irrespective of whether the hemiplegia was a product of damage either to the right or the left hemisphere. In fact, there was right hemiplegia in 21 cases and left hemiplegia in 23 cases. However, those patients who during infancy develop hemiplegia associated with the dominant hemisphere after speech has developed, lose speech for some months, but then it returns and eventually they speak quite well. Although speech may have formulated itself in association with one hemisphere in these cases it is still possible should that hemisphere become damaged to employ the other hemisphere for this purpose. Obrador (1964) also reports little speech disturbance following hemispherectomy in infantile hemiplegia patients, and indeed, on occasion, an improvement in speech output was to be observed. Hodgson (1967) confirmed this and his patient spoke in a normal voice with good articulation and there were no observable differences in speech or language following hemispherectomy.

When damage occurs to one hemisphere only early in life there is little or no language loss following adult hemispherectomy of either side. When, however, the adult experiences a rapid invasion of pathological tissue in one hemisphere and no evidence exists of severe damage early in life the picture is very different. After right hemispherectomy there may be no speech impairment and only moderate or little impairment on verbal tests (Mensh et al., 1952; Rowe, 1937). After excision of the left hemisphere there is considerable language disturbance (Gardner et al., 1955; Hillier, 1954; Zollinger, 1935). Gardner et al. (1955) argue that parts of the brain cannot 'take over' functions as easily in adults as in children. Speech laid down in one hemisphere is affected in tumour cases by removal of the dominant hemisphere and the other hemisphere in the adult is unable to substitute.

Smith (1966) and Smith and Buckland (1966) report observations on a case of left dominant hemispherectomy for glioma in a 47-year-old male. Standard test batteries were used to provide evidence on both the initial and later effects on language and non-language functions. The subject was right-handed and right-eyed before left hemispherectomy. Right hemiplegia followed the surgery. Although lacking the dominant hemisphere this patient surprisingly had some residual mainly automatic speech but his speech was still severely impaired 13 months post-operatively in spite of the fact that he showed some recovery of verbal comprehension as well as some ability at reading and writing. His comprehension was impaired but not grossly so but he remained severely aphasic. It should be said that it is difficult to infer much from this case because the patient died from a tumour recurrence this time in the right hemisphere two years post-operatively and it is not clear how this affected right hemisphere function.

When cases of infantile hemiplegia are considered the evidence suggests that each hemisphere has considerable potential at first to take up the speech functions. In the case of the adult brain the situation is more closely defined. Interference with speech shows a close association with left hemisphere damage, whereas speech may remain unaffected following right hemispherectomy. (The residual speech in the case described by Smith remains something of a puzzle.) A clear distinction must be made between speech and language. Speech represents the final link in the language chain and is governed by an output system. Interference with the output system will result in a disturbance of speech. At the same time it cannot be assumed that this implies a complete loss of potential for expression of linguistic capacities through means other than speech. Although we may suppose speech to relate to one hemisphere it is necessary to exercise caution. We cannot say that linguistic potential is also the exclusive province of that same hemisphere.

It has been remarked that the infant can part with his cortex with less resulting functional disturbance than can the adult. Adult language is exceedingly complex. More time may have to elapse in order for the remaining hemisphere to take up an advanced and complicated function than a relatively simple one. It does not follow that the adult brain has a total loss of functional plasticity.

HIGHER MENTAL PROCESSES

Rowe (1937) reports, in one of the first observations on hemispherectomy, that the patient succeeded remarkably well on tests of verbal intelligence. This led Hebb (1959) to remark 'that the patient incredibly succeeded with tasks that would baffle 80-85 per cent of the normal population—making it certain beyond question that a new base of operations was needed for study of the relation of brain to intelligence'. Previously the concept of mass action had held wide currency. This relates intellectual functions to the total amount of brain tissue available. It follows from this view that a man with only one cerebral hemisphere should be at a profound disadvantage. The case cited by Rowe showed little if any of the impairment which was to be expected. It seems to be the case that a remarkable preservation of abilities is generally to be observed following hemispherectomy.

A variety of reports exist in the literature concerning intellectual functions. Griffith and Davidson (1966) showed in studies made before and after hemispherectomy of twelve surviving patients at an interval after surgery averaging over ten years, that a significant gain of intelligence was to be observed in five of the twelve patients, whereas six other patients showed slight but insignificant gains. It is in those whose injury was at birth or in the first year that a gain in intelligence was noted. These were cases of infantile hemiplegia and presumably the deteriorated hemisphere, far from being inactive, exerted a negative influence on the functioning of the other. Hodgson (1967) also reports in the case mentioned previously of a 17-year-old girl that before surgery this patient had a WAIS verbal I.Q. of 64, and a performance I.Q. of 49, providing a full-scale I.Q. of 55. After the operation this patient showed improvement. Her verbal I.Q. rose to 79, her performance I.Q. to 75, providing a new full-scale I.Q. of 76. There was, in addition to this change on the intelligence score, a marked improvement of behaviour. Ueki (1966) reported, however, that one or two months after surgery there may be a fall in test scores, whilst an improvement occurs one or two years later.

Smith (1966) and Smith and Burkland (1967) carried out a variety of tests on the patients they studied following hemispherectomy. Those with right hemispherectomy with the exception of one who showed mild language defects were well within the normal range as measured by the intelligence test used. Sub-tests of the intelligence scale used as a test of concept formation and generalizing ability or the capacity to abstract important principles indicate that capacities involved in verbal abstract reasoning were not noticeably impaired.

However, patients with right hemisphere removal showed subnormal performance on items which reflect visuo-spatial and visuo-constructional functions, visual memory and non-verbal analogous reasoning. Jackson (1874) described the left hemisphere as 'leading' in language and he considered the right posterior lobe as leading in the visuo-ideational processes. The performance of the three patients with right hemispherectomy supports the view of an association of the right hemisphere with visuo-spatial functions, but here again care must be taken to analyse the exact nature of the association in order that an exaggerated picture of lateral differences is avoided. None of these patients showed any evidence of psychosis, bizarre behaviour, or impairment of volition or will (Smith, 1969). None revealed the deficits described in cases of restricted lateralized lesions. The picture of intellectual function following hemispherectomy may well be different from that after more restricted lesion. This suggests that remaining tissue can exert an active but often deleterious effect. Such tissue may have potential for recovery of something approaching normal function, whereas absent tissue cannot show this but in cases of hemispherectomy the potential rests exclusively in the capacity of the remaining hemisphere.

McFie (1961) examined the case histories of 34 patients. The time of onset of brain injury showed itself to have an important influence on the results. If the hemisphere was damaged during the first year of life, patients showed a significant increase in intelligence test scores following hemispherectomy. There was no difference between right and left hemispherectomy. It seems reasonable to suppose again that the damaged hemisphere is having a deleterious effect. McFie (1961) points out that many patients return to average levels of performance on intelligence tests following hemispherectomy in cases of infantile hemiplegia, and that those patients do not usually exhibit E.E.G. abnormalities in the remaining hemisphere. The fact that patients produce intelligence scores within the average range post-operatively, shows that in some people at least a high degree of normal function is preserved, and that the single hemisphere in cases of this type is sufficient to mediate most of the activities the individual is called on to perform.

Possible changes in integrity and balance of the individual's personality are an important topic for investigation. Some authors suggest that hemispherectomy makes little if any difference to the way an individual behaves (Griffith and Davidson, 1966; Smith and Burkland, 1966; Smith, 1969). Others suggest that prior personality problems, temper tantrums, rages, being difficult to handle, etc., may well improve following hemispherectomy (Carmichael, 1966). Improved behaviour and progress in the development and structural formation of the personality has also been reported by other workers in follow-up studies of patients examined several years post-operatively. Personality development as revealed by projective and intelligence tests may be virtually normal and it is reported that 'the young patient is in many cases able to carry on a satisfactory social and scholastic life. He can take part in normal activities and earn his living.'

Other investigators, however, report deteriorative changes. Gardner et al. (1958) suggested that undesirable personality changes are the sequelae of hemispherectomy. They suggested that their patients become dependent and regressive. Bruell and Albee (1962) also report personality changes in a hemispherectomized patient. This patient was a 39-year-old man who developed a tumour in the right fronto-temporal area. On intelligence tests he showed a remarkable preservation of intellectual function four months post-operatively. His Wechsler Verbal I.Q. was 121 and his performance I.Q. 76. However, he began to show a distortion of the time sense, and a lack of concern about future events. The patient, although impotent, became uninhibited and increasingly preoccupied with sexual matters. However, he developed a tumour in the remaining hemisphere, and it seems possible that at least some of these disturbances could be attributed to this cause.

Evidence of personality disturbance was also presented by Osson (1966) in a study of twelve hemispherectomized patients. Osson suggested that the patients show motor hyper-excitability, a tendency to automatic reactions and rapid exhaustion following more demanding actions. Emotional excitability was evident, and also it is suggested some disorganization of temporo-spatial structuring.

There are many difficulties in evaluating possible personality changes following from a surgical procedure such as hemispherectomy. The patient may show bizarre or disturbed behaviour before surgery. The pathology causes disturbance and it is for the relief of this that the surgery is undertaken. In addition, there may be secondary anxieties and frustrations which follow in the wake of the pathology as the result of the circumstances in which the individual finds himself. Patients after surgery may show temporary euphoria because the operation no longer hangs as a threat over them. Apart from these difficulties associated with pathology, there are other difficulties in assessing personality changes. Standardized techniques can be used, but these are not yet developed sufficiently to provide a high degree of objectivity. Judgment as to whether a change has or has not occurred may be suspect because different investigators use widely different yardsticks. Then again, one investigator may emphasize the importance of some changes, other investigators the importance of others. In view of these difficulties and the fact that the reports in the literature do conflict, it is necessary to proceed cautiously. It would appear that much of personality organization can be preserved following hemispherectomy, although the possibility must be encompassed that either facilitative or deteriorative changes can follow as a consequence.

The problem of consciousness has been a persisting one. Recently it has been the subject of considerable speculation and review (Burt, 1967; Sperry, 1966). Hemispherectomy can throw some light on this problem even if it is of a limited nature. It is possible, for example, to ask such questions as 'does the patient experience a loss of consciousness following hemispherectomy?' or 'does one hemisphere hold the monopoly of conscious experience?'.

In response to the first question, it is often the case that disturbances of body consciousness accompany hemispherectomy. Usually these are temporary and disappear rapidly during recovery. Bruell and Albee (1962) report the case of a 39-year-old man who had hemispherectomy for glioma. Post-operatively he had a left hemiplegia with a disturbance of body consciousness on the left side. During the first few days the patient refused to acknowledge his paralysed left side. When he was made to touch his left hand or leg he insisted that the hand or the leg belonged to someone else. This symptom, encountered frequently in patients after damage to the right cerebral hemisphere

(Weinstein and Kahn, 1955), subsided after a period of approximately three weeks. He was then able to localize stimuli at the left side and body image was described normally. There may be a loss of conscious experience with regard to the contralateral side but this is essentially temporary. At no time could it be said that the patient lacked conscious experience of the right side, or that he lacked consciousness in general.

Wada and Rasmussen (1960) developed the technique of intracarotid injection of sodium amytal. This test was performed on two hemispherectomized patients by Obrador (1964) to study the effects of functional inactivity of the residual hemisphere. The intracarotid injection of 200 mg of 10 per cent sodium amytal solution was made on the side of the remaining hemisphere. The patient showed an immediate loss of consciousness which lasted from four to six minutes. The patient is functionally decorticate and following the temporary loss of function of the remaining hemisphere, subcortical activity was released. Flexor or extensor rigidity of the limbs was followed by automatic mass movements. A passive movement in one of the limbs induced a series of continuous and repeated automatic movements which persisted for some time. The responses patterns were those of bilaterally decorticate individuals.

In none of the cases reviewed here is there evidence of a loss of consciousness from hemispherectomy. Consciousness or the alert state of the brain is not destroyed by the removal of one cerebral hemisphere. Where hemispherectomy takes place under local anaes-thesia there is no loss of consciousness even immediately post-operatively. This is true of right or left hemisphere removal. Despite reports to the contrary (Eccles, 1965), it is certainly not the prerogative of only one hemisphere to possess consciousness. Whatever the nature of consciousness it is clear that it exists in both hemispheres and that each is capable of operating in the alert state.

CONCLUSIONS

The surgical removal of a cerebral hemisphere provides important evidence about brain function. A remarkable fact in cases of infantile hemiplegia is the degree to which one hemisphere can stand in for the other. Where there has been early brain damage, much of the capacity lost from one hemisphere is restored by the other.

The loss of a major portion of the brain may not totally incapacitate a patient. Bruell and Albee (1962), for example, on meeting a patient in the fourth month following hemispherectomy were surprised to find 'a man who could discuss his condition in a seemingly detached and objective way'. Smith *et al.* (1969) reporting on a case of almost total atrophy of one cerebral hemisphere, with chronic infantile hemiplegia and displacement of the remaining hemisphere into the midline position, state: 'This patient reveals remarkably good mental and physical development considering the magnitude of her cerebral anomaly.' Statements of this kind indicate that the functional deficit may belie the not unreasonable expectation that profound disturbance will follow hemispherectomy. Indeed, the evidence led Hebb (1959) to suggest that a new base of operations was needed in the study of the brain.

Hemispherectomy and unilateral lesion in animals provides evidence that each hemisphere is capable of resuming most of the major functions of the other. There is no substantial reason to think that a permanent relationship establishes itself, whereby one hemisphere directs the functions of the other, and as far as can be ascertained, the functional relationship is a cooperative one with considerable overlap and duplication of function.

The human brain in very early life presents a not dissimilar picture. At this time one hemisphere appears to be largely capable of substituting for the other. With regard to electrical activity, the removal of one hemisphere does not lead to permanent disruption of the other's functions. Instead the remaining hemisphere rapidly adjusts to the fresh demands which are made upon it. With regard to motor function, patients who develop cerebral pathology in one hemisphere early in life are not greatly affected by removal of the other, and up to a certain age potential exists both for relearning and for transfer of motor functions from one to the other. Also, in cases of infantile hemiplegia, the existing hemisphere appears to have the capacity to monitor and control the perceptual processes which ordinarily would be present in the hemisphere which has now been removed.

With regard to speech, each hemisphere has at first a potential for speech development so that if gross damage occurs at an early age in one hemisphere, all speech processes will be transferred to the opposite hemisphere. The adult may not retain this potential and speech will then become the specialized function of one hemisphere. In cases of infantile hemiplegia there is a remarkable preservation of intellectual function following hemispherectomy, and the fact that consciousness persists suggests that it is the exclusive prerogative of no one hemisphere.

Evidence of this kind lends support to some views of hemisphere interrelationships more than others. Results from animal studies and some of those from hemispherectomy in cases of infantile hemiplegia and early damage to the human brain emphasize the similarities between the two hemispheres. For example, after either right or left hemispherectomy patients show no disturbance of consciousness and in many cases preserve a remarkable degree of intellectual functions. This does not accord with the theory that one hemisphere unchangingly dominates and directs the functions of the other.

As for the view that function is distributed unilaterally either to one or the other hemisphere, this can only be supported in so far as speech and visual-ideomotor tasks reveal a greater deficit following the removal of one hemisphere than of the other. Nevertheless removal of one hemisphere still leaves a considerable residue of performance in the other and it may be unwise to assume that one hemisphere has unique responsibility for a particular function. Integration of activity may well play a part in the organization of a function even though that function may appear to be related more to one hemisphere than the other.

Studies of hemispherectomy point irrevocably to one central conclusion, that one hemisphere either replicates or has the potential to replicate the functions of the other. It seems highly probable that in a duplicate system of this type, cooperation between areas is the rule rather than the exception, and the results of studies suggest a tandem as well as a duplicate system in which each partner may have a share in the direction and control of behaviour.

6

The Double Brain and
Concepts of Skilled Performance

INTRODUCTION

Studies of skilled performance have exerted a profound influence on the way we think about both brain function and the organization of human behaviour. Much of their impetus derived from the early work of Bryan and Harter (1897, 1899) who investigated the twin skills of morse key tapping and typewriting. Whilst primarily concerned with the acquisition of skill and charting the progress of the person under training, these studies also posed the problem of how it is possible to carry out complex tasks at all. What must be the nature of the brain organization which enables a complex sequence of acts to be put into operation? How is it that the person is able to send the correct message, or type the correct response in relation to the information received? In its complexity, range, and accuracy, this represents a remarkable capacity as any person who has attempted to model the same by construction of artificial analogues will testify.

These early studies also developed a method by which the performance of an individual could be subjected to analysis. This method was the check-list technique which measured performance by comparing, in the case of typing, what has to be typed with what actually is typed. The information so to speak, passes from the printed page into the typist's brain, and then back once more, through the action of her fingers, to the page. By comparing the original text with the final product, it was possible to assess the typist's accuracy;

There have been many such studies since, comparing input with output and these led Craik (1948) to the view that the brain could be regarded as similar to a computer calculating the odds and using them to produce a lawful output. Views of this kind were amplified and given fuller treatment by Weiner (1948) in his discussion of cybernetics, and by Shannon and Weaver (1949) and their followers in studies of mathematical theories of communication. More recently the same impetus has been at work in studies of decision-making as expressed in theories of signal detection (Tanner and Swets, 1954; Swets, 1964).

One feature arising from this view of human performance is the interest that has centred on the upper limits of capacity. Experimentation has been directed at assessing exactly how much information can be dealt with over prescribed limits of time. Hick (1952) attempted to define the information capacity of the human operator. Welford (1952, 1967, 1968) studied the capacity of the human operator to deal with two signals one shortly after the other, and Broadbent (1958) the capacity to deal with more extended simultaneous messages.

The original investigations of the decision processes were based on the assumption that the brain acts as a channel of limited capacity. Needless to say, the view of brain function as a single decision system is something which runs counter to the arguments presented here. Therefore it is essential for us to review ideas of single channel brain function in the light of later evidence which suggests first that the hemispheres function together, and secondly that they possess some capacity for independent analysis of incoming information. This does not mean that single channel limitations do not operate at some points in the chain of analysis, merely that they do not apply along the whole route of the sensory-motor system. The evidence put forward to support this view is that of the author's own investigations, as well as much additional experimental work which shows that brain capacity exceeds that predicted from a simple single channel view. Evidence is also quoted to show that decisions can be made at the same time as the channel is occupied in processing information which has already been received.

REFRACTORINESS AND RESPONSE BLOCKING IN THE CEREBRAL HEMISPHERE

Bills (1931) began a study of blocks to function and showed that the prolonged performance of a colour naming task resulted in occasional slow responses of twice the value of the mean response times. Bills called these slow responses 'blocks'.

Intermittent failures have also been observed on vigilance or watch keeping tasks whose characteristic feature is that the person has to look for infrequent signals over long periods of time. Mackworth (1950) for example required the subject to watch the movement of a pointer around a clock face. The pointer jumped in a regular fashion from one position to another but occasionally it would jump a double length, and the task was to detect this. Failures appeared with increasing frequency as the subject continued the task. These have been attributed to central nervous system origins (Broadbent, 1956).

This type of failure is characteristic on tasks with infrequent information performed over protracted periods of time. Examples in the everyday work situation are radar watching, and inspection tasks where the observer detects flaws in a completed product. Another block to performance occurs in the refractoriness situation. Here the subject is asked to respond to two signals one occurring very shortly after the other. Although response to the first signal is completed in the usual time, response to the second signal may be delayed. Increase in response to the second over that to the first has been described as a psychological refractory period. The concept of refractoriness is by no means new in the study of nerve function and it has a strict application. It describes the lack of excitability and conductivity which follows the appearance of the nervous impulse (Samson Wright, 1965).

The spike potential leaves the nerve totally unresponsive to fresh impulses and is said to be absolutely refractory. During the next few milliseconds strong stimuli can arouse the response although weaker stimuli fail to do so. The nerve is now said to show a stage of partial refractoriness.

The concept of refractoriness has been applied perhaps incautiously to nervous functions on a larger scale. It is used not only to describe the block to function in a single nerve but also the block to further function in the brain after the passage of a signal which has been received and is in the process of analysis.

Bertelson (1965) reviewed the evidence for this and described it as central intermittency. Typically response proceeds to a first signal but response to a second signal arriving a few milliseconds after the first is delayed. Welford (1967) argues that the delay is a function of the limited capacity of the human brain, and he supposes that it reflects the operation of a single channel mechanism.

The concept of the single channel does not fit with the evidence in the preceding chapters in support of the view that the brain is an effective bilateral mechanism; evidence that each hemisphere has some capacity to remember, to learn and to perceive as well as to control and direct behaviour. If there are two independently functioning perceptual systems it may be asked why there should be any delay to a second signal? Could not one hemisphere analyse the first and the other simultaneously analyse the second? The answer seems to be that yes, they can, and as we shall see later if each of the two signals is lateralized to a separate hemisphere then delay is considerably reduced. The idea of refractoriness is compatible with the view that there exists more than one system for analysis of incoming information. There are several points to be considered here. One is that it takes time to arrange a transfer of information from one hemisphere to the other. Also the hemisphere may find that it needs to analyse incoming information before making a decision to allocate it to the other hemisphere, thus a second response will be delayed. It may be that delay to the second signal represents nothing more nor less than the time taken to distribute the load between the cerebral hemispheres.

In the non-lateralized condition because the same sequence enters both hemispheres, the hemispheric system employing each member alone or in conjunction with the other, will take as long to analyse the material and organize response as it would if only a single channel operated in the brain. The two views therefore are not incompatible but there is more to the question than the minimal time to function. Total capacity may not be revealed by this. For example it takes only as long to play a recorded message on a single tape recorder as it does to broadcast that same message over a major radio network, yet it would not be denied that the latter has the greater capacity.

There are other considerations which lead us to support the bilateral hemisphere view. Elithorn and Barnett (1967) describe experiments in which they suggest that normal subjects respond independently to stimuli presented to opposite visual half fields. Information lateralized in this way is projected to only one cerebral hemisphere. The results suggested that each hemisphere takes up information and organizes response in a way which may well not be directly dependent on the functions of the other.

The subjects were shown a central warning light; this was followed by a visual signal to one or both visual half fields. The subject was required to press a response key as quickly as possible with the corresponding hand. Stimuli occurred either alone or in pairs, one at each side. The results suggest that in many subjects independent processing of information is possible at each hemispheric locus. Presumably at some stage in the complex chain of events leading through from signal to response, each hemisphere acts independently of the other to code and classify the information it receives. If the argument is put forward that each contains its own perceptual analysing mechanisms, than it should be possible to determine the limits of perceptual load which each can take as well as to show that the use of two hemispheres as receiving stations is better than the use of one. Two hemispheres should provide a greater capacity when their functions are combined than when they are employed separately. These possibilities led the present author to begin a study of the cerebral hemispheres as perceptual analysing systems to assess their capacity to deal with information and to study their efficiency as receiving centres both separately and independently (Dimond, 1969a, b, 1970b, c).

It was clear that considerable potential existed in the method of directing signals not to the centre field of vision but to either the temporal or nasal retina, thus projecting them to separate cerebral

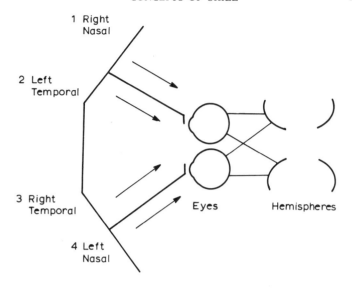

Fig. 13. Diagram of apparatus and visual pathways.

hemispheres. If reaction time tasks were given using this visual arrangement the possibility arose of timing the response after the signal had entered one hemisphere, and comparing the speed of that response to that when the signal enters the other hemisphere, thus it should be possible to compare the relative efficiency of each. The possibility also existed of timing the transit of information from one hemisphere to the other by providing information to one and demanding response from the other.

The first investigation* undertaken with these objects in mind was one of simple forms of reaction time. In previous experiments information had been directed towards the centre field of vision, i.e. the information from the display was projected to both hemispheres. No difference had been discovered in the response times of one hand and the other. The average response times of the hands were of a similar order, and did not differ significantly. The averages concealed the fact, however, that one hand tended to lead the other, but the left hand led as frequently as the right, and there was no tendency for one to lead consistently in preference to the other (Dimond, 1968, 1970d). If one hemisphere leads in the speed of its functions the response of its hand

* The author is greatly indebted to the Medical Research Council for their support which enabled the investigations described here to be carried out.

should be made first. The fact that this was not so led to some questioning of the established ideas of cerebral dominance in relation to hand function (Dimond, 1970a). The next task was to lateralize the perceptual information more closely, to confine it to a particular hemisphere and to test response from each hand to signals projected to different hemispheres.

The perceptual display was similar to that used by Gazzaniga (1965) to study split-brain patients. Signals were projected either to the right or to the left of a central fixation point. The task was to react to each signal as quickly as possible. Signals were projected to only one half retina at a time. This is illustrated in the accompanying diagram. A signal was projected to any one of the hemi-retinae, and the subject's task was to respond as quickly as possible using one hand. The subject performed with one hand first and then switched half-way through to the other hand. Although information was strictly lateralized to one hemisphere or the other, there were no differences in the response times between one hand and the other (Dimond, 1969a). It would seem from these results and those examining response to different kinds of stimuli (Dimond, 1970c), that each hemisphere may be as effective as the other in the organization of relatively simple responses. Each appears to possess the capacity to organize, control and trigger, simple response patterns and furthermore each appears to take a roughly equivalent time to accomplish this.

These studies of simple response times to only one signal revealed little, if any, difference between the functions of one hemisphere and the other. Studies were then undertaken of each hemisphere's capacity to deal with two signals arriving at the same time. These revealed various blocks to efficient function. The subject received the two signals simultaneously, not one immediately after the other as in the traditional refractoriness experiments (Dimond, 1963, 1970c). These experiments form part of a large body of recent research, which examines the person's capacity to deal with two or more streams of concurrent information.

Broadbent (1958) reviews his own investigation of function when two series of digits are directed simultaneously to different ears. In other experiments by the same author series of digits were presented to the ear, and the other series to the eye. Kimura (1961b) adopted and extended the use of this method to the study of brain damaged patients. It has also been used to study the effects of division of the cerebral commissures (Milner *et al.*, 1968). In relation to these investigations there are a number of questions which need to be posed. What happens when the brain is required to deal with two signals arriving at the same time when these are both signals for response? What will happen when signals for response arrive together at the same hemisphere? Will one hemisphere be more efficient than the other? When concurrent signals arrive at different hemispheres will the use of two hemispheres as receiving stations prove to be superior to the use of one? Needless to say if it were possible to answer questions of this kind we could throw light on the problem of whether the brain is organized as a single channel or if the numerous neurological investigations which suggest an inherently duplicate or tandem system could be confirmed.

In an experiment by the present author (Dimond, 1970c) two signals at a time were flashed to the subject. These were arrows pointing either to the right or the left. An arrow pointing to the right was a signal for right-hand response, an arrow to the left a signal for left-hand response.

The subjects of the experiment responded to a series of different arrow arrangements. On one trial they were shown one arrow alone, on the next they might see two arrows pointing in different directions. They were thus not able to predict what the next response was to be. The divided visual field method described previously of projecting signals to particular hemispheres was used and it was found that when two signals are projected to the same hemisphere there is a considerable block to the performance of response. It can be seen from the accompanying figure that response times are considerably extended when both stimuli are projected to the single hemisphere.

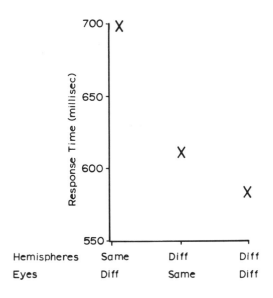

Fig. 14. Response times to two signals flashed at the same time, either both to one hemisphere or each one to different hemispheres.

There is also a block to function when two messages are passed through the same eye. Some mutual interference exists at this level, but this is not our primary concern at the present time. The fact that interference exists between the response to messages at the hemisphere level indicates something of the limitations of function of each cerebral hemisphere as an information system. Interference between one message and another when these are directed to the same hemisphere indicates that disruption of the essential processes for analysis of the messages is taking place. The question can now be asked, why does the hemisphere not simply unload its burden and pass the signals to the other hemisphere for analysis? This would liberate the one receiving hemisphere from the load imposed upon it. The answer seems to be that the one hemisphere is not able to do this because the nature of the nervous arrangements within the brain constrain it to analyse its own information before sharing with the other can be encompassed. In other words, stimuli are not only received but they also enter the analysing system of that hemisphere which processes them in an exclusive way before contact for load sharing with the other hemisphere takes place.

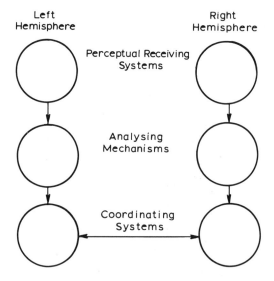

Fig. 15. Diagram to show that perceptual information is analysed before coordination with the other hemisphere occurs.

Thus interference arises because two messages of a conflicting kind have entered the one analysing system of the same hemisphere and act mutually to disrupt the process of their analysis.

Mutual interference operates on both sides of the brain, i.e. interference occurs whenever both messages are directed together to either one of the right or the left hemispheres. There is some evidence that the right hemisphere shows more interference than the left, but this question will be taken up at a later time. Mutual interference between messages is a characteristic feature when the messages are directed to a single hemisphere.

So far in the discussion of these results it is possible to suggest that mutual interference is a characteristic of brain function as a whole and that the direction of messages to the single hemisphere exemplifies this general principle. If, however, we refer to the results again, we find that if one message is directed to one hemisphere at the same time as the other message is projected not to the same but to the opposite hemisphere, then the same degree of mutual interference does not occur. Messages directed to separate hemispheres are dealt with more effectively than two messages directed to the same hemisphere and the same blocks to function are not now to be observed. These experiments support the work of Elithorn and Barnett (1963) who suggested that independent processing was a possibility. The results also show that the picture obtained from split-brain patients has important corollaries in normal human function. Further than this they point to the need to study the perceptual systems of normal people in the light of duplicate brain mechanisms and the possible tandem arrangements operating between them.

Whilst the results demonstrate that mutual interference occurs between messages when these are projected to the single hemisphere, it might be argued nonetheless that if the effect is to be described as refractoriness it is necessary to show that the passage of one message into the system has effects which last and act upon subsequent messages directed shortly afterwards to the same system. In unpublished experiments it was possible to show first that if one signal was directed to one hemisphere and the second signal directed to the other, there was little if any delay in response to the second signal (Dimond, 1970a). If, however, one signal was projected to ,one hemisphere and the second after a delay of 100 milliseconds to the same hemisphere, either the right or the left, then response to the second signal was considerably protracted and delayed. This result again suggested that independent analysis proceeds in each cerebral hemisphere, and that limits to analysis appear in the single hemisphere condition. These results suggest also that whilst one hemisphere is analysing a particular message there will be a delay before it becomes free to analyse another subsequent message, although such analysis may be achieved by the opposite hemisphere.

Mutual interference can be illustrated yet again in experiments

DB—5

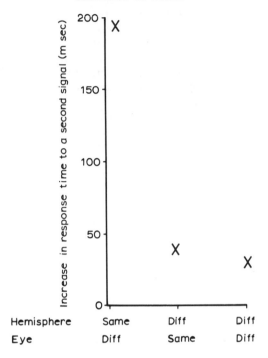

Fig. 16. Increase in response to a second signal following the first after an interval of 100 ms.

which employ verbal material (Dimond, 1970a, 1971a). Letters were projected on to a screen in front of the subject. Four letters projected in sequence comprised a word. The subject was shown two of these series of four letters making two words at a time. His task was to say what the words were, or failing that as many letters of each word as he could remember. The subjects commonly reported one word and perhaps a few letters of the other word. When one word was projected to one hemisphere and the other word to the other, the percentage of words correctly reported increased. When, however, both words were projected to the same hemisphere the number of words accurately reported showed a decline. Blocks to function are again observed. When both words are projected through different halves of the same eye there is a deterioration of performance. However, disruption is much greater at the hemisphere level and when both words are projected to the same hemisphere there is an even more marked decline. Once again stimulus material at the same hemisphere is mutually disrupting, showing the limitations of the decision mechanism of each hemisphere; indicating

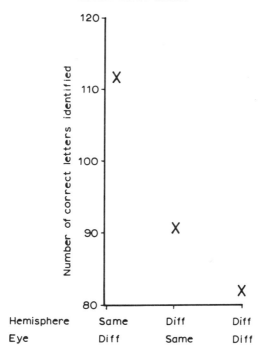

Fig. 17. Number of letters reported correctly: two words flashed at the same time, either both to one hemisphere, or each one to different hemispheres.

also that these same limitations are not to be observed when the messages are directed one to one hemisphere and the other to the other. This supports the view that two systems operate in the brain at the hemisphere locus, each capable of a degree of independent function and each apparently working to analyse material before sharing the burden of information load with the other hemisphere.

Another method to assess capacity is to require the individual to perform two tasks at the same time (Dimond, 1966). If in an overload situation of this kind the signals of one task are projected in such a way that they are shared between the cerebral hemispheres this should lead to an increase in the total capacity of the brain which will be reflected in the amount of task that the individual can perform. Using the apparatus described previously, subjects reported digit pairs presented at the rate of one per second (Dimond and Beaumont, 1971). Each member of the digit pair was either projected both to the same hemisphere, or one digit of the pair was projected to one hemisphere,

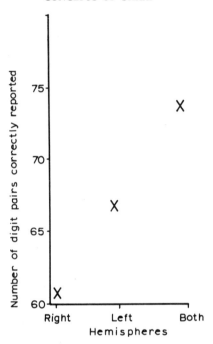

Fig. 18. Score on visual task performed in conjunction with sorting task. Signals projected to the left, right, or both hemispheres.

the other member to the other. At the same time the subject sorted nuts and bolts into two bins using both hands, out of sight below the apparatus but conveniently within reach. Although the results on the sorting task failed to reach significance, when the visual task was distributed between the hemispheres significantly more digit pairs were correctly reported than when the visual task was projected to a single hemisphere.

It has been shown therefore that when perceptual load is distributed between the cerebral hemispheres, total output is increased. This result provides further confirmation that each hemisphere possesses its own perceptual analysing system and ,that each acts as an information channel, while the use of two information channels proves itself superior to the use of one. The presence of two analysing systems showing parallel activity creates the possibility of distribution of the perceptual load between conjoint systems, which is apparently a characteristic mode of brain function not only in split-brain patients but also in normal individuals.

LATERAL CONTROL AND RESPONSE COMPATIBILITY

It has been suggested in earlier chapters that organization for lateral control is a pervasive feature of the brain. This arose presumably in association with bilateral symmetry. Not only is it necessary for the brain to deal with laterally distributed events in external space, but also to organize responses of the body in relation to them. Even in primitive organisms there may be an advantage in rapid spatial identification and tagging of events from the right and the left and in the capacity to associate lateral events with corresponding lateral arrangements of the motor system. In human behaviour we find that the need to coordinate and phase in responses with events occurring in space is a very real one. Although central vision and the movement of the eyes towards central field material ensures the use of both hemispheres, nonetheless, signals which identify stimuli as being of potential importance frequently come from the periphery of vision. In these cases one cerebral hemisphere only is stimulated, and this sets the response to the stimulus in motion, whether it be the focusing of the eyes directly towards the stimulus, or the immediate reflex to a danger signal. The double system separates out stimuli coming from the left and those coming from the right. It differentiates the spatial direction of signals and permits rapid directional response to be made without delay or confusion. The system operates on inherent separation by virtue of the separate anatomical nature of the hemispheres.

Craik (1948) suggested that the fundamental feature of neural machinery is its power to parallel or model external events. This is true with regard to left-right discriminations and evidence is available of a special relationship between the lateral position of signals and the corresponding responses made to them. Blyth (1963) for example, examined confusions which arise between the responses of the limbs when the response of one is requested a short period after the response of another. The greatest number of errors was found between the hand and foot on the same side of the body. Extended response times occurred in this situation. In other words, when two responses are required from the same hemisphere, response blocking occurs, reaction time is extended and response of one may be substituted for that of the other. This argues for inter-dependence in the organization of responses relating to the same hemisphere as well as independence between one hemisphere and the other. Blyth (1964) confirmed that the responses which interfere most are the ones organized from the same hemisphere. Rabbitt (1965) also reports that the greatest delay is experienced between the limbs on the same side of the body. This supports the view of the brain as a paired system in which each member has the capacity for analysis of incoming information to some degree independently of the functions of the other, and a system which shows limitations and blocks to function which previously have been thought to typify the whole brain but which now seem to relate more specifically to the functions of each single hemisphere itself.

It is now our task, to examine more closely the way in which stimuli occurring either to the right or to the left in space become related to corresponding response patterns. In a task described by Welford (1958), the subject was required to rotate a steering wheel to keep a pen centred upon a moving track. Movement of the wheel to the right moved the pen to the right. This was a 'natural situation', and high levels of performance were achieved. Steering which worked the other way round, however, caused great confusion, i.e. wheel moves to the right but the pen moves to the left. Reversed control relationships are difficult to manage and the subjects make numerous errors (Griew, 1959). The most natural relationship of making a movement to the right to conform to the movement of the display to the right appears as a built-in arrangement which Welford (1968) describes as the 'mark of skill akin to the extraction of constants'. The subject can learn to move the wheel to the right when the display moves to the left, but performance is inefficient and there are tendencies to revert back to the more 'natural' movements (Welford, 1968). This can be regarded as a natural consequence of the existence of an anatomical through route for perceptual information from one side to relate to motor response of the same side. Griew (1958, 1964) used a task in which the subject was required to move a stylus from a centre point. Signal lights were placed just behind the targets. In some conditions the subject was required to aim for the target on the opposite side to that signalled by the stimulus light. This was a highly incompatible situation. Not only were response times slow, but response times increased even more sharply if there were a large rather than a small number of alternatives.

Broadbent and Gregory (1967) also report a refractory period experiment in which the task was made difficult by requiring response to the right stimulus light to be made with the left hand and the left stimulus light with the right hand. One stimulus followed a short duration after the other. Response to the first signal was extended as expected on the basis of making an incompatible response. Not only was response time to the first signal increased but response to the second signal was even more protracted, taking on average 800 milliseconds. The second reaction was delayed when the second stimulus arrived after the first response has been completed and it is clear that a residual effect remains from the passage of the first response. This could reflect the time taken through the use of cross talk to sort out which hemisphere is to be employed in the analysis of each signal and the organization of each response. It may be expected on these grounds that the difficult stimulus response relationship in Broadbent and Gregory's experiment would lead to response times to second signals which are considerably protracted. The results could also be viewed as related to hemispheric competition. Stimuli occupying the spatial position to the left not only enter the right hemisphere but call for response from the left, and vice versa. Both hemispheres are maximally involved and rivalry and inter-hemispheric competition may occur. A response using an unusual and unfamiliar relationship creates a greater after-effect than an established one.

It is not surprising that the special anatomical system for separate analysis of information from the left or from the right should reflect its activities in performance. The organism uses paired receptors to differentiate events in space and the brain is an internal extension of this system. It is to be expected therefore that the cerebral hemispheres play a natural part in the analysis of spatial function. The hemispheres could be regarded as a mechanism for rapid segregation of stimuli from different regions of space. It seems reasonable that the brain should designate each hemisphere to proceed with the analysis of the information exclusive to itself before at some later time the input from both left and right are integrated and combined. Whatever the nature of the comparison, the brain provides for immediate spatial analysis in having two hemispheres which act separately to a large extent in control of lateral body functions but also differentiates in anatomical representation between left/right events in space. The experimental results on compatibility of stimuli and response make manifest the effectiveness of these systems for coordinating lateral stimuli with lateral response.

CHANNEL CAPACITY

Each cerebral hemisphere has some independent capacity to register and analyse the information which influxes into it. If information is directed to one hemisphere at the same time as some is directed to the other, then two hemispheres are better than one in accuracy and amount of the end product. It is essential, however, that each receives information concerned with a different portion of the task. These results foreshadow a picture of brain function as a tandem arrangement involving each hemisphere in the analysis of its own information but allowing provision nonetheless for the two to coordinate their activities by a continual cross-talk.

The pathways from major sense organs to each cerebral hemisphere are duplicated and most of the time each hemisphere will be in receipt of common information. Scope for independent action may be restricted and this may give the impression of a unitary output. The appearance of unitary function cannot always be used as an argument that duplicate channels do not operate. A bottleneck to the transmission of information at the stage of the selection of motor response for example will impose severe limitations on the the whole system. Again, although each hemisphere may show independent analysis of incoming information a bottleneck where the coded information from each hemisphere is integrated will also impose severe limitations upon performance. Limitations operate at certain points in the chain of nervous command, but at the same time it cannot be argued that these necessarily apply to the whole chain or that every link is subject to their control. We would particularly wish to argue that the prior and antecedent links do not work under this influence.

Evidence for the single channel view can be obtained from a number of sources. Craik (1948) noted in studies of tracking, that the person behaved as an intermittent correction servo. The subject was required to trace a track using a pencil. If the track moved the subject was required to follow it, just as a gunner might follow a moving enemy target. The person following the moving target failed to show a smooth response, but instead tracked with a series of corrective movements jerking in a backwards and forwards fashion, movements being made at discreet intervals of half a second. Craik concluded that these results show something of the limitations of the central mechanisms of the brain. He supposed that the results could not be due to the limitations of the motor mechanisms because hand movements of the extent and nature required could be made much more quickly than the required two per second. The fact that motor movements can be made quicker under different circumstances is not necessarily an argument that the delay does not arise from the motor system. Be that as it may, Craik (1948) suggested that the delays in responding are due to the 'time-lag' caused by the building up of some single computing process.

Subsequent studies by Vince (1948, 1950) required the subject to keep a pointer on a line drawn on a paper band which passed behind a narrow slit. At intervals the line abruptly changed position and the subject's task was to follow these changes as closely as possible. When the need arose for two changes to be made close together in time, the second change was delayed sometimes by an appreciable period. This led Welford (1952) to suggest that only one, or at least one group of signals at a time, can be dealt with by the central decision mechanism and thus he formulated the single-channel view as a theory of the psychological refractory period.

Davis (1956) modified this theory somewhat but broadly stated it holds that the second reaction time is lengthened by an amount equal to the interval between the arrival of the second signal and the end of the first reaction. Only after the completion of the analysis of the first response can that of the second begin. Not all authors report this effect and Brebner (1968) for example, found that the delay to the second signal may not always occur as for example in the processing of signals conveying instructions to continue a responding movement.

The theory of the single-channel has been developed by Welford in further papers (Welford, 1967, 1968) but the single channel view is not the only theory of the decision processes of the brain. It has been suggested, for example, that parallel information processing more closely fits the observable facts. We shall return to this view which is the one emphasized in this chapter, but first we have to discuss the single channel view in more detail.

A bottleneck to the transmission of information not necessarily a motor one can occur at any one point in the complex chain of neural events leading from the stimulus to the response for results to be produced which would favour the single channel hypothesis. Perceptual analysis could proceed in a variety of parallel systems, and yet restrictions could be superimposed which to all respects limit the operations to single channel functions.

It is not the purpose here to question that results are obtained which support the single-channel view under the circumstances in which it has usually been studied, or that the results point to some limitation of function at whatever stage of the system this applies. The study of the refractory period is however a special case whereby the person is constrained to respond as rapidly as possible to the advent of signals which normally he cannot predict. In other words, he responded to a situation likely to expose the temporal limits of his performance. The temporal limits of performance need not however reflect the capacity of the system as a whole and if care is taken to restrict visual input to one hemisphere rather than another, a different picture emerges.

The facts are that two signals directed to the single hemisphere set up a mutual interference and when the second signal follows the first by a short delay, response to the second signal is delayed. These effects are not observed when one member of the stimulus pair is projected to the other. In other words, each hemisphere possesses its own limited 'central' decision mechanism. Furthermore, whilst each shows this same effect, some of the limitations do not apply when both the decision mechanisms of each hemisphere are employed on the same task.

These results do not support the view that the brain operates as a single channel of limited capacity. They support the view that each cerebral hemisphere acts as a decision mechanism, and that both together are capable of working in parallel to enhance performance. In summary therefore, although the brain may be regarded as a single channel system, it seems reasonable to suppose that it acts this way in only part of the chain leading from the initial stimulus to the production of response, and that indeed the cerebral hemispheres have some capacity for independent analysis prior to response organization. Each hemisphere is a single channel limited capacity system, and there are two systems and not one system of this type in the brain.

THE CEREBRAL HEMISPHERES AND INFORMATION PROCESSING

It has already been proposed that the results which support the concept of single-channel operation can refer to any bottleneck of the system, and that what may be typical of this region need not apply to the system as a whole. The possibility for parallel processing at one stage is not incompatible with the view that single-channel operation exists at another stage. It has been suggested however that parallel systems for the analysis of information exist one in each hemisphere, and that the brain is a double system.

Another source of evidence concerns the capacity of the brain to act as a communication channel in the more rigidly defined terms prescribed in the mathematical theories of communication (Shannon and Weaver, 1948). Communication networks consist of a transmitter, a communication channel and a receiver. Information may be coded before entering the communication channel and decoded at the receiver. In comparing the quantity of information emerging from the receiver with that entering from the transmitter, the efficiency of the system as a communication channel can be prescribed. Some information may be lost, there may be inclusions and distortions but this simple comparison allows a useful estimate of the information carrying capacity of the channel.

Investigations of human behaviour have employed similar although not as readily quantified methods since the beginning of scientific studies of behaviour. The subject is presented with materials and his response to these is tested. Thus in a memory experiment the subject is provided with items which he memorizes and subsequently he is tested for his retention of those items. The information is given to the subject who is the communication channel and is recovered from him by the experimenter. It was not long before the concepts of mathematical communication theory were applied to this situation, indeed studies of this kind have experienced a considerable vogue during the past two decades. At this present time enthusiasm has waned, and fresh areas are being pursued, but the legacy of this approach remains, and the value of regarding the brain as one of this category of systems is still apparent. If the brain is regarded as an information system, then it may be expected to use a binary code. The binary code allows the most efficient transport of information. The greater the quantity of information to be transmitted the longer the time it would take. In fact, for each additional quantifiable bit of information, an additional constant period of time will be required. The time taken to respond therefore increases as a straight-lie function of the amount of information to be transmitted, assuming that channel capacity is limited and that information is processed in a binary fashion. Broadly speaking, this was confirmed by Hick (1952) who predicted that the greater the quantity of information to be processed the longer it will occupy the channel. Hick required subjects to respond to signals selected from a different number of choices. As the number of possible signals increased, so response time increased in relation to the amount of information. Several other investigators have also shown this. The amount of information is defined technically as the probability of a signal occurring from a specifiable number of alternatives (Bricker, 1955; Crossman, 1956).

Hick's law, as it has been called, relating the time of response to the number of alternatives, has been extended to other situations. Crossman (1953) for example, required the subject to sort playing cards into different categories, working as quickly as possible without making errors. The number of classes into which the subject was required to sort, varied from one trial to another. He might simply sort red cards from black; on another occasion he may be required to sort by suit, or by number. The results appeared to confirm Hick's law that the greater the number of classes the longer the time required for the decision. This is not the time or the place to report in detail on either the history of information theory or on its more recent developments. The reader interested in pursuing this line of inquiry is referred to Attneave (1959) and Edwards (1963).

There have been many critics of information theory. It has been said that the person establishes a subjective criterion as to the number of alternatives from which stimuli may be regarded as being drawn and the external measure of the number of alternatives may not correspond with the situation as the subject sees it. This criticism is particularly relevant in the light of the developments in modern decision theory. Other criticisms are that the temporal sequencing of information may act to facilitate or interfere with the final end-product of the information. If, for example, the responses should become out of phase with the information transmitted at the signal source, then information transmission may break down with disastrous results for the skill (Dimond, 1963). These criticisms, pertinent as they are, are not our main concern at the present time however, because the more important problem of the limits of human function have yet to be discussed.

Evidence has accumulated which suggests not only that human performance may not correspond to the predictions laid down in Hick's law, but that it can, on occasions, transcend that which is predicted as possible. Although for much of the time the person behaves as a limited capacity channel, and a single channel at that, he may not always do so. A model more closely fitting the situation would be one of two or perhaps more decision mechanisms, each showing limitations, but each acting in parallel with the other.

Circumstances which reveal the capacity to process information beyond the limits prescribed by the single channel theory are those where a high degree of stimulus-response compatibility is achieved and those where the responses of the subject are already highly practised.

In the first place we have already seen that the slope of the curve for the rate of gain of information depends on the compatibility or otherwise of the stimulus and the response, i.e. in situations in which the subject finds difficulty in pairing the stimulus and the response the slope of the curve becomes exaggerated (Crossman, 1956; Griew, 1958, 1964). Treisman (1965) also showed that the accuracy with which subjects could repeat either English or French words showed only a small decline with increased speed. Or one could say, the subjects were processing increasing information per unit time. There was, however, a considerable drop in efficiency when the subjects, bilingual subjects at that, were required to translate from one language to the other.

Leonard (1959) found that when subjects responded to vibratory signals administered directly to the responding finger (i.e. the signals and response are as compatible as possible) no evidence was found of increasing response time with increasing numbers of alternative stimulus response pairs beyond the two-choice conditions. There was no further increase in response time either in the four- or the eight-choice condition. In information theory terms an eight-choice situation represents a greater information load than a two-choice situation. Furthermore, if the view is accepted that the central decision mechanism is limited to a single channel, then *ceteris paribus* it should be impossible for reaction times in the eight-choice situation to be the equivalent of those in the two-choice situation. Brainard *et al.* (1962) also report high rates of information transmission when a familiar set of signals (numbers) was paired with the familiar response of speaking and repeating back the numbers. The number of choices from which the signals were drawn proved to influence the results minimally in this condition, although this became a more significant factor with less compatible stimuli and responses. Leonard (1959) was inclined to attribute much to response compatibility and supposed that if the relationship between the signal and the response was wholly compatible, then the slope with increasing numbers of choice remains at zero.

Leonard's results were not the only ones to cast doubt on the view of the brain as a mechanism processing information through a single channel. When responses are highly practised, response times for high numbers of choices can be brought down to that of a two-choice situation.

Mowbray and Rhoades (1959) and Mowbray (1960) showed that with sufficient practice response times in the ten-choice situation can equal those in the two-choice situation. Pierce and Karlin (1957) also found that reading time was closely similar whether words were selected from vocabularies of 16 or 256 common words. This again shows that with familiar material response times may be far faster at high levels of choice than the theory of the single limited capacity channel would lead us to predict.

Davis *et al.* (1961) also found response times to be much shorter than was to be expected for items chosen from a large number of alternatives. These authors played nonsense syllables recorded on tapes to their subjects who were required to repeat each syllable as quickly as possible. At first the time taken to repeat back syllables chosen from the larger set was greater than that for the smaller set, but with practice the two-choice time remained the same, but the times for the four and eight choices diminished considerably. Knight (1967) also examined the effect of practice and found that response times for higher degrees of choice were all markedly reduced after practice.

Garner (1969) reports experiments in ,which the subjects were required to sort cards into two packs. Two alternative stimuli provided the feature critical for the sorting, but in addition a variety of redundant features were included, such as the distance between dots, the orientation of dots, etc. The cards were sorted faster with these additional features and it was argued by Garner that this is due to the capacity of the person to process the information serially rather than sequentially. These results strongly suggest that where a high degree of stimulus response compatibility is a feature of a task, and where an opportunity exists for the responses to become well practised, the human subject easily transcends the limits for information processing which might have been predicted on the basis of the view that the individual operates as a single channel.

Stimulus response connections may become so well established that they are ready for use on each trial rather than available only after a lengthy process of search and analysis. Another alternative view is that the brain has the capacity to carry out informational analysis in parallel. The evidence of the preceding chapter suggests that parallel processing is a feature and there seems little reason to deny the possibility of such. The work described by the present author shows that performance may be enhanced if the information load is shared between one hemisphere and the other. It seems reasonable to think that the capacity for parallel processing asserts itself even on tasks in which the separation of input to each cerebral hemisphere may not be distinct.

In the case of highly compatible responses differentiation of input to each hemisphere may be a feature of the task arrangement. In the experiment described by Leonard (1959) the vibration of an armature stimulated the finger that was used to make the response. In fact, a close correspondence existed between the stimulus and the responding member. There is almost complete lateral representation of the sensory system in the cerebral hemisphere; the left body surface in the right cerebral hemisphere and the right body surface in the left. The hands are controlled by the contralateral hemisphere although some ipsilateral projection exists. The most complete representation within the same hemisphere of both the stimulus and the response occurs in compatible stimulus response relationships. The compatible situation is one which utilizes the double processing system most fully and it may well be this which leads to efficient response. In highly practised responses, the subject is able to predict the processing demands. He could exercise a strategy to distribute the information load between the hemispheres, thus invoking their tandem arrangement and provide scope for an increase in information handling capacity.

SELECTIVE PERCEPTION

The capacity to select some items to be perceived but not others has received emphasis in recent years. It is well known that some stimuli never capture the attention mechanisms. The person reading an interesting book may remain oblivious to conversations held simultaneously in the same room. There have been numerous experiments of selective listening which require the subject to listen to two simultaneous messages. This work has been summarized by Broadbent (1958). The object of these experiments was to examine the response to simultaneous messages and the subject commonly responds to one message but ignores the other.

Some of the first results were obtained by Cherry (1953). One message was played to one ear at the same time as another message was played to the other. The subject repeated back only the message played into one ear. Practically nothing could be reported subsequently of the message on which is known as the rejected ear, i.e. the ear receiving the unwanted message. If a change of language occurred or the speech was played backwards in the message to this ear, the subjects failed to notice. Broadbent (1958) in an attempt to explain these results, postulated the presence of a filter which acts to block off unwanted messages. Broadbent (1952a, b, c) found that when two conversations arrive simultaneously over a loudspeaker, the subjects experience difficulty in listening to the messages because one message interferes with the other. However, the confusion between the messages is not an inevitable function of just receiving two spoken messages because if the voices speaking the messages differ in their physical qualities they can be distinguished reasonably well. Differentiation between them is not as difficult if one message is spoken by a man's voice and the other by a woman's (Broadbent, 1952b). It is also the case that the messages can be differentiated more readily when one conversation is louder than the other or when one has the lower frequencies removed (Egan *et al.*, 1954). The messages are more easily registered also if the two voices emerge from separate loudspeakers arranged in a position one on each side of the subject (Poulton, 1953). There are also lateral separation effects and Hirsch (1950) reported that speech was easier to hear in noise if the loudspeakers producing the noise were placed on the opposite side to that producing the speech, or when speech occurred to one side whereas the loudspeaker producing the noise was placed in front.

These results indicate that when there is a differentiation according to physical characteristics, there is a much clearer separation of the messages. They indicate also that the physical separation of the sources is an important feature and that when the speakers are placed on either side of the individual, the messages are easier to comprehend. Taking the early results of Cherry (1953) as they stand, and viewing them from the framework of the auditory functions of the cerebral hemispheres, there are several considerations to make. The contralateral projection fibres are relatively more massive than the ipsilateral ones. The indications are that primary projection of auditory material occurs to the contralateral hemisphere. If at the same time the ipsilateral pathways acted to block the functions of their own hemisphere, the contralateral hemisphere would be available exclusively for the purpose of the analysis of the message, and here we might expect the rejection of other material. Alternatively, it may be that messages, whilst primarily directed to the contralateral hemisphere, are also funnelled through the ipsilateral pathways to the ipsilateral hemisphere. The message is received, in this case at both hemispheres. It would be expected that mutual interference would occur with each message, but they would interfere less with one another to the extent that they were tagged by physical characteristics such as the speaker's voice or the spatial separation of the stimulus sources. These factors could act as aids to prevent the mutual interference which, on the basis of the hemispheric refractoriness studies, we might have expected to come about. The question now has to be asked as to how it is possible to attend to one message and ignore the other. Licklider (1948) showed that in listening to speech in noise, hearing was easier when the speech message was in phase and the noise was out of phase. Two spoken messages to the extent that they differ, appear inevitably as a series of events which are to a large extent out of phase with one another. Although the word lengths are matched there will still be differences of emphasis, time and style unless resort is made to synthetic computer speech (Haggard, 1970). Under these circumstances, the subject may differentiate one message from what is effectively a very noisy background, but the task of differentiating the two messages would be beyond the capacity of the individual. This may be possible however where aids were provided to increase the degree to which the messages can be discriminated and to increase their dysphasic nature as occurs with spatial separation of the sources, or the use of male and female speakers. The message chosen for report would appear to depend on which one was easiest to differentiate from the other, and which one the subject had been instructed to reproduce.

The picture which emerged from the first results showing that one message totally excludes the other is one that has not been wholly confirmed by subsequent investigations. Treisman (1964) used two messages and played one to each ear. The subject found it easier to concentrate on one message rather than the other, but when a message came to one ear whilst at the same time another message was played to both ears, or alternatively two different messages were played to each ear and then in addition to that, a third message was played to both ears, and it was more difficult to reject the unwanted messages. This suggests that when a message is lateralized primarily in the one hemisphere, it is easier to exclude another message. When, however, both messages use the primary pathway to the same hemisphere, this same separation is no longer as effective and mutual interference is characteristic. This is equivalent to ,the hemispheric refractoriness noted as a feature of capacity to deal with visual information. Once again, the physical features of the auditory message play a crucial part because in control experiments employing rhythmic repeated sounds, separation of the wanted and unwanted messages was relatively easy in all conditions.

Occasionally words from the unwanted message break into the wanted one if they are particularly appropriate to the context (Triesman, 1960). When the subjects were required to switch halfway through an experiment from one ear to the other, a few words from the wrong ear often broke into the reported message, the subject not realising that they had done so.

Moray (1959) repeated Cherry's experiment. He included the subject's own name in the unwanted message and found that this would break through into the reported message. This suggests that some analysis of the data proceeds in conjunction with that of the spoken message, although the unwanted message may subsequently be rejected. Then again, Peterson and Kroener (1964) found in their studies that whilst retention of the secondary message was poor, it was by no means the all or none affair that Cherry reported. Some items at least from this message could be recalled.

Investigations have subsequently been undertaken to determine the extent to which information is retained when it occurs in a second message which is not spoken or shadowed. Lawson (1966) required the subject to shadow a message on one ear and to ignore the message on the other. A series of 'pips' were played to either ear and the task was to press a key at the left when a pip was heard on the left ear, and a key at the right when a pip was heard on the right ear. Substantial numbers of correct responses to pips were made, although they occurred on the unwanted channel. This indicates that the unwanted channel is not completely neglected and that total exclusion of material on it does not occur. Although the perceptual mechanisms are occupied with the analysis of one message, nonetheless at the same time analysis is proceeding of the messages on other channels.

Abrams and Bever (1969) also present evidence which is at variance with the channel view. They provided the subject with clicks which required response whilst he was reading a twelve word sentence. Reaction time to clicks located between the clauses of the sentence were not the fastest ones as might be expected and they suggest that the channel view might be appropriate for that part of the speech process which occurs after the immediate organization of speech into segments but not otherwise.

Lawson (1966) suggests in relation to her experiments, that analysis of physical signals precedes both a selective filter as well as those mechanisms concerned with the analysis of verbal content. Triesman and Geffen (1967) also suggest that selection is made before the full analysis of the verbal content of a message. In their experiment they required the subject to speak aloud, one of two messages but at the same time to tap if a word belonging to a particular class was represented in either the shadowed or unshadowed message. Some facility for this was shown when the word was included in the unshadowed message, although naturally enough, performance improved if the word was included in the shadowed message.

Further investigations were made in which subjects were required to listen for letters in either ear and to stop shadowing a given message at once and tap with a ruler (Treisman and Riley, 1969). More digits were detected in the ear they were shadowing (76 per cent compared to 33 per cent) when the target letters were spoken in the same voice as the digits, but when the letters were spoken in a different voice and could be distinguished more easily by their physical characteristics the subjects detected almost all of the letters on both ears. This suggests that a filter operates not to block messages totally as the results of Cherry suggest, but to attenuate them whilst other messages are in progress. There is much evidence to support the view that secondary messages are in fact attenuated (Broadbent and Gregory, 1963; Webster and Haslerud, 1964; Yates, 1965). At the same time the finding reported by Moray that a subject may respond to his or her own name suggests that unused input can be scrutinized and inspected before being relegated to the category of unworthy for further analysis. Not only can the subject deal with one stream of information and organize responses in relation to it, but at the same time additional processes work to sift and segregate information although it may not be necessary to proceed further with its analysis. The work of Lawson, and Triesman and Geffen, suggests that analysis of incoming information takes place at a stage antecedent to that of more detailed inspection. Exactly what characteristics are used in this is difficult to say. It is a matter of importance that there are antecedent systems in the chain of perceptual analysis. It is not clear however that the idea of a mechanism of preattention differs substantially from that of separate analysing systems which function on one side to preserve the chain of message to response but at the same time use another system to differentiate features of additional messages.

Each hemisphere receives a projection from the contralateral and the ipsilateral ear. A message is most strongly represented from the contralateral ear and is perceived against the background of ipsilateral interference. In the dichotic listening situation therefore the message from one ear is most strongly represented in the contralateral hemisphere and the second message in the other hemisphere. If both messages have similar properties the brain may only differentiate one of the two messages, both hemispheres being employed on this; the one chosen depending upon the instructions given and other factors.

In an easier situation each hemisphere may analyse the message transmitted to it in spite of interference. It will scrutinize the perceptual information relevant to the wanted information, and set the response train in motion to the message. The second hemisphere not receiving the direct influx of the wanted message could also be employed for the greater part in the analysis of that message, this second hemisphere, however, has the unwanted message projected to it at full intensity through the massive contralateral fibres. The second hemisphere is in a unique position for the prior scrutiny of the unwanted message. Each hemisphere can to some extent proceed independently with the analysis of perceptual information, and a distinct possibility exists, to place it at no higher level than this, that the hemisphere hearing the unwanted message scrutinizes it to ensure that nothing of significance is missed.

The full equation has yet to be made between dichotic listening studies and hemisphere functions. There is however good evidence of independent analysis by each hemisphere. The wanted message could be scrutinized by one and the unwanted message by the other. It is not necessary to suppose that analysis must or can only occur through attentive and a preattentive mechanism linked in sequence.

CONCLUSIONS

Although there are bottlenecks to function within the brain, this chapter suggests that these limitations may not operate along the whole chain of decision by which the subject receives information, analyses it, and uses it for response. Recent investigations suggest that each hemisphere has the capacity to analyse information in its own right, and that when information is shared the capacity of the brain is increased.

Experiments in which two signals or two streams of information are projected to the same hemisphere show that a block to function exists which interferes with the full expression of response, i.e. each message interferes mutually with each other message. This may indicate that the characteristics of limited capacity, formerly ascribed to the brain as a whole, are best ascribed separately to each cerebral hemisphere.

Mutual blocking and refractoriness of messages projected to the single hemisphere suggest that analysis occurs within the hemisphere to which the information has been projected and that there is apparently no overspill into the other hemisphere. Each hemisphere cannot escape the responsibility of analysing the information which enters it, nor can it unload additional information to the other prior to analysis. This suggests that each contains an analysing system which, along part of its length at least, functions independently of the system operating in the other hemisphere. At present then this system appears to have the characteristics of a single channel, but in time it may well be proved capable of a higher degree of analysis.

The view expressed here is that the results supporting the picture of the brain as a single channel provide evidence only of a bottleneck to the transmission of information. They do not rule out the probability that each hemisphere acts as an analysing system and that duplication of function is a feature of the chain of nervous control. Indeed, evidence for this is available from the author's own studies, from studies of the rate of information processing, from studies of lateral response compatibility and from studies which show that some analysis of unwanted messages occurs in the dichotic listening situation.

7

Laterality

INTRODUCTION

The paired arrangements of the more advanced animal brain appear, with few exceptions, to be totally symmetrical about the central body axis. The physical features of one half of the brain match those of the other, and when the functions of each are mapped, each appears to form the mirror image of the other. A more or less complete matching of function between right and left hemisphere is the rule for species lower than man in the phyletic scale. This characteristic feature of the brain as an organ balanced and duplicated in its function represents a basic design of the nervous system.

When we consider the brain of man we have to ask to what extent he also conforms to this typical pattern. Physical examination reveals symmetry and duplication around a central body axis. There are reports of physical asymmetries, but frequently these come within the normal range of variation and are not statistically significant. The physical picture of the brain as we know it today is one of an almost completely lateralized and duplicate system. When we consider function, we observe a different picture. Some of the similarities between one half and the other have been passed over, and differences emphasized at their expense. Nonetheless differences do exist.

HANDEDNESS

One obvious difference is the movement patterns of the limbs. This is most commonly thought of as handedness, but differential preferences also apply to the use of the lower limbs and to the use of one eye rather than the other. There are other aspects of body function, e.g. facial expression, to which the concepts of laterality apply. Sutton (1963) for example, found a relationship between a person's handedness and the position their nose occupies on the face. There is also evidence for somatic effects. Wolff *et al.* (1964) report consistent differences in the perception of superficial and deep somatic pain between the right and the left hand. Weinstein (1963) also reports that discrimination between a single and a two-point threshold may be more accurate on the right body surface in right-handed patients.

There are some reports of paw or hand preferences in animals. Usually the animal performs a task which permits only the use of one hand, for example to reach through a hole to obtain an item of food. If it consistently employs the same hand then it is said to show a preference for the use of that hand. Consistent although weak and obscurely defined ,preference for the use of one paw rather than another occurs in mice (Collins, 1968) and rats (Tsai and Maurer, 1930; Peterson and Gucker, 1959; Peterson and Vine, 1963). In general most animals show a high degree of ambilaterality, i.e. either paw may be used to secure food objects, but some animals, a smaller proportion, show a preference for the use of either the right or the left paw. The number preferring the right is usually the equivalent of those preferring the left. A similar situation applies in the case of the cat (Cole, 1955; Warren, 1958) and monkeys may show little preference on easy tasks, but a more definite preference on difficult ones (Kounin, 1938). The number of ambilateral animals consistently outnumbers those showing preference (Ettlinger, 1961, 1964; Hall et al., 1966; Warren, 1953; Milner, 1969). Generally the proportion of animals showing a preference for the right is the equal of that showing a preference for the left (Finch, 1941; Cronholm et al., 1963).

When the lateral preference shown by human beings is considered we find a different position. There is a marked preference throughout the population for the use of the right hand. Groden (1969) reports that 81 per cent of normal schoolchildren are right-handed, and only 6 per cent left-handed. In the adult population the number of left-handed people may be less than that. However, the division of the population into two categories, right or left-handed, may not represent the true state of affairs. Gillies et al. (1960) described how certain subjects who wrote with their left nonetheless preferred to use the right hand for certain other actions. They suggest that the mixed-hander is a basic biological variant. Problems have arisen because of a failure to distinguish possible mixed from pure cases. Annett (1967) presents evidence for the value of recognition of this category. Groden (1969) following Annett's classification, reports that 13 per cent of the population of schoolchildren are true mixed-handers. In evolutionary terms two important factors emerge, one is that the large majority show a preference for the use of the right over the left, but the second is that whilst the number of representative mixed handers is small they still form a significant proportion of the population.

It may be that left/right differences become apparent from the first days of life. Turkewitz et al. (1963) report differences in head turning responses to left and right localized stimulation of the perioral region in three day old human neonates, finding more ipsilateral and fewer contralateral responses to right than to left stimulation.

Other writers regard lateral preference as developing much later, Travis (1931) for example, states that strong consistent hand preferences do not characterize younger children. Washburn (1929) and others, also commented on the relative symmetry of the movements of the extremities in infants. At first the responses of one limb appear not to be closely differentiated from the other, and the movements which do occur are those of the paired structure as a whole. Gesell and Ames (1947) suppose that asymmetrically differentiated responses arise subsequently out of originally bilaterally integrated movements. Several authors also have described the instability of the initial asymmetrical movements, and the fact that they may be submerged by the symmetrical bilateral patterns.

There is evidence also to suggest that asymmetry in motor function is associated with other aspects of developmental status. In view of the notoriously difficult problem of assessing this in an accurate and meaningful way however, caution must be taken in the interpretation of the results. Cohen (1966) reports that 43 per cent of eight-month-old babies prefer the use of their right hand whereas, by comparison, 90 per cent of their mothers prefer to use the right hand. Cohen reports that those babies who show a marked preference for the use of a particular hand were more advanced than the others, and that such a development may be considered an effective way of dealing with the environment, but this may be a parallel development. Dreifuss (1963) also reports that whilst speech as well as hand dominance are not delayed in children having sustained a lesion in one or other of the cerebral hemispheres, even a mild bilateral deficit does not affect the development of speech and handedness.

Although the use of one limb in preference to the other emerges as characteristic, somewhat older children may still show a marked degree of ambilaterality. Belmont and Birch (1963) state that the younger age groups are more ambilateral and left/right discriminations also follow a developmental course. In relation to this Wapner and Cirillo (1968) report that at first the child shows a large proportion of mirror image responses when attempting to copy the movements of another person but progressively over time transposition occurs and the child responds instead with the limb on the same side as that used by the experimenter.

Some authors have taken an environmentalist view supposing that cultural factors are of great importance. Falek (1959) for example, observed that left-handed fathers produced fewer left-handed progeny than expected, and he suggested that the fathers were influential in changing the hand preference of the children because they themselves found it a disadvantage to be left-handed. Other authors support a view based on the genetics of handedness. Annett (1964, 1967) supposes that handedness is determined by two alleles, D which manifests right-handedness and R which manifests left-handedness. D is usually dominant and R recessive, but there is also a partial penetrance of R in heterozygotes. Annett shows that this model fits data on the distribution of handedness in the population. There seems good reason to support a belief in a model of this kind, and although such a model may not be an exact fit, nonetheless the binomial distribution appears to account remarkably well for the facts.

There have been reports of either a greater incidence of ambilaterality or left-handedness in certain clinical or psychologically disturbed groups. The exact significance which attaches to these reports is difficult to assess. In some cases difficulties are ascribed to mixed laterality or a high degree of ambilaterality, but at the same time it is not at all clear that there may not be some associated anomaly or disturbance of brain function which is responsible both for the behavioural difficulty and the pattern of laterality which the person may show. Differences in the pattern of laterality may be slight and of marginal and not of great statistical significance, and care has to be taken not to read too much into results which can perhaps be accounted for in other ways. For example, many of the early reports suggest a higher incidence of left-handedness in stutterers, epileptics, and those people showing reading disabilities (Hildreth, 1949a, b). This same finding has been reported for mental defectives (Murphy, 1962; Jones et al., 1967). The factor responsible could well be localized brain pathology acting to displace hand preference away from the affected hemisphere, and leading to a more even distribution of hand preferences amongst these groups. The reported relationship between reading disability and handedness may also relate to similar pathology at least in some of the groups studied (Dearborn, 1933; Orton, 1937; Benton, 1959).

There is evidence that the motor skill of the hand may be impaired by appropriately sited lesions. Ghent et al. (1955) showed, using 36 patients with unilateral penetrating brain injury, that normal learning of a tactual discrimination problem occurred with the ipsilateral hand, but learning with the contralateral hand was severely impaired. This investigation emphasized the importance of the hemisphere which receives the principal projections from the stimulated surface. Benton and Joynt (1959) in a study of response time in brain damaged patients, found also that all brain damaged patients were slower than controls, but at the same time there were specific unilateral effects to be observed, although no evidence existed of clinical motor deficits. Evidence supports the view that brain damage can lead to differences in lateral preference. Wyke (1967) reports that in normal subjects the speed of single arm movements and of alternating repetitive movements is faster using the right than the left arm. A left-sided lesion reduces the speed of the arm contralateral to the lesion, as well as slowing somewhat the response of the ipsilateral limb. Right-sided cortical lesions slow the movements only of the contralateral arm. These effects are most commonly associated with lesions of the parietal region. Wyke (1966) showed, in a test situation in which the subject was required to maintain a static posture of the extended arm in the absence of vision, that patients with parietal lesions show significant degrees of arm drift and that a left-sided lesion produces impairment of both the contralateral and the ipsilateral limb, whereas right-sided lesions produce postural impairment on the contralateral side only. Wyke (1967) also reports in a study of pursuit rotor performance that the right arm was significantly better than the left, and that in subjects with unilateral lesions, impairment of performance occurred in both the ipsilateral and the contralateral limbs, but if care was taken to exlude patients with visual field defects, performance deficit related only to the contralateral limb in patients with right-sided lesions, but remained bilateral in patients with left-sided lesions. This reflects the greater proficiency of the right-hand over the left for the performance of various tasks by right-handed subjects. It has also the implication that the left hemisphere plays a greater overall part in performance control than the right and this is a question to which we shall return later.

Although the preferred hand is obviously the superior in many respects, this superiority may not be reflected in every measure of performance. Ojemann (1930) noted that handedness varies with the nature of the activity studied and he pointed out the significance of the fact in playing the violin or another comparable string instrument that the difficult and dextrous job of fingering is accomplished by the left hand in right-handed players. Oldfield (1969) using his own sinistrality index, took up this problem. It seemed remarkable to him that the left hand should be employed in this complex work and he thought it possible that there may be a higher proportion of left handed people who are musicians. In fact, neither more nor less musicians were left-handed than the undergraduate population at large. Oldfield suggested that in spite of the use of the left hand for this task, right-handedness is less a matter of superior inherent dexterity or the capacity for agility precision and speed than the more immediate availability of the right hand as the instrument of the individuals conceptions. The use of the left hand by the violinist for fingering should however cause some reflection before it is supposed that the differences between the performances of the two hands are as absolute as we might otherwise believe.

Studies of handedness more often than not are concerned with preference rather than measures of strength or skill. Where attempts are made to measure other factors the differences may not be as striking. Simon (1964) studied steadiness, handedness and hand preference. The subjects classified themselves with respect to handedness. They performed a steadiness task with one hand and then with the other. Performance was somewhat better with the preferred hand, but not outstandingly so, and Simon states that hand steadiness cannot be regarded as a sensitive index of handedness. Even amongst people who strongly typify themselves as left or right handed some task may be performed better with the non-preferred hand and the relation between skilled performance and the handedness which a person reports may be far from perfect (Benton et al., 1962; Satz et al., 1967; James et al., 1967). Kimura and Vanderwolf (1970) also report that isolated flexion of a single finger is not executed better by the preferred hand, and that rather the data for right-handers at least indicates the opposite. Kimura and Vanderwolf suggest the superior performance of the left in making individual finger movements may be due to greater pryamidal innervation to that hand and, of course, the relationship to fingering in violin playing is relevant to this finding.

When other factors such as pressure sensitivity of the palms, soles of the feet and forearms are considered then right-handed subjects may show greater sensitivity at the left, and left-handers a greater sensitivity at the right, paradoxical though it may seem. (Weinstein et al., 1961). The over-riding preference for the use of one hand rather than the other need not imply superiority in all functional respects. In many cases this will be so, but with the exception of writing and possibly drawing the functions of one hand match, or at least fall not far short of those of the other.

Some non-preferred hand functions equal those of the preferred hand after practice. The pianist, for example, may achieve equal facility with the left as with the right hand. The concept of learning limits has been discussed by Ferguson (1954, 1956). He suggests that the choice of hand relates to over-learned performance by that hand. There is a possibility that the non-preferred hand could be trained to the same level. In this context Provins (1967) concluded that there may be little or no difference in relative performance on tasks which involve only simple movements, but that significant differences occur when more complex serial organizations of muscle movements play a part.

In simple tests of muscle strength (Roberts, Provins and Morton, 1959) and accuracy of the reproduction of pressure (Provins, 1956), no difference between the sides may be recorded. Competent typists required to type with either the right or the left hand showed no differences in accuracy or speed, whereas non-typists showed better performance with the preferred hand. With practice, the non-preferred hand had improved in competent typists to equal the performance of the preferred hand (Provins, 1967). Perhaps hand functions are not governed by fixed limits but have at least some potential for change?

The small differences in response times between one hand and the other have generally failed to reach appropriate levels of statistical significance (Benton and Joynt, 1959). Dimond (1970c) in studies of visual response time in the hemispheric situation, confirmed the view that simple response times of the hands may not differ although information has been directed to either the right or the left hemisphere. This conforms with the view expressed by Provins (1967) that differences between the hands are unlikely to be observed in respect of simple movement patterns.

Dimond (1970d) studied performance when both the right and the left hand are required to respond at the same time. Two stimulus lamps close to each other provided signals to the subject. Visual input was not in this case separated out to each hemisphere. The left light was a signal for left hand response, the right a signal for right hand response. At first response was made to either the right or the left signal, but subsequently both signals, the right and the left, appeared together. Response was required with both hands. In this situation the right competes with the left for first response and superiority of the preferred hand should be reflected in its capacity to win out over the other. One hand responded faster than the other and the first hand tended to respond at an interval of one response time before the second. However, the one responding first was by no means always the right hand. The right hand could win and it did so on some occasions but only as frequently as the left. The chance was a 50/50 one that either would lead the other in the speed of its functions. Hand responses seem to be organized on an either/or basis, i.e. one response emerges first, but at the same time the first response can be that of either the right or the left. The apparently equiprobable nature of this system ensures that one response, and presumably one only, is available to the situation, be that the response of either the right or the left hand.

These results could perhaps be explained by reference to a centrencephallic movement system organizing response patterns at a level below that of the cortex. There is evidence for subcortical involvement in the organization of motor patterns. The cortex may instruct that courses of action are to be pursued without at the same time spelling out in detail the plan for their finer organization. Instructions from either the right or the left cortex could enter a system which acts to order and structure but not to initiate the pattern of movements. A system may carry out the serial ordering of behaviour, but even so, cannot be envisaged as the only process involved. Before impulses finally emerge to set up the patterns of muscular activity, they could themselves process through sub-organizing systems, specific to each side of the body, and it is these which become progressively more involved with increasing complexity of the response.

This model is one of many which could be suggested in an attempt to understand the workings of the motor system. Models tend to be descriptive of the events which they are supposed to explain and this is no exception. All that is claimed is that this model may help in thinking about the problem of motor control.

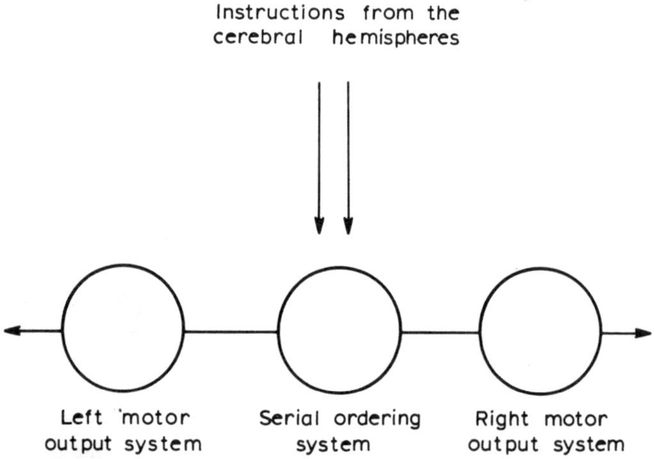

Fig. 19. Hypothetical model of a system for the ordering of motor output.

The next task is to discuss the relationships which the facts of handedness have to hemisphere function. The traditional view holds that the hemisphere which relates to the preferred hand is the one which predominates in its functions. Taken to the extreme the argument holds that one hemisphere overshadows the functions of the other; it dominates and directs, whereas the other is subordinate. It may be that a simpler explanation can be provided.

The facts of handedness are not substantially open to doubt. The evolutionary course has taken man towards asymmetry of hand preference. Yet at the same time we must beware of a tendency to suppose that handedness is an all or none affair. There are different degrees and complexities of laterality.

Some authors suggest that lateral differences can be explained by differences in the speed of neural conduction between the hemisphere and the limb. One hand functions more effectively than the other because the speed of impulses transmitted to it by way of the motor nerve is that much faster. Right-handed subjects show faster conduction velocity in both the right ulnar and right median nerves than in the left ulnar and median nerves, whereas left-handed subjects show a faster conduction velocity in both the left ulnar and median nerves than in the right ulnar and median nerves (Cress *et al.*, 1963). Other results could support a similar interpretation. Efron (1963) found that a delay is necessary when stimuli are delivered to each half of the body separately (2-6 milliseconds) in order that the stimuli be perceived as simultaneous. Cernacek *et al.* (1967) also report when recording from the parietal region of the scalp, that after stimulation of the ulnar nerve the early response occurred first more often in the dominant than in the subordinate hemisphere, although no difference was recorded in the late response.

Much could be explained by differences in the speed of nerve conduction between the brain and the hand in either the sensory or the motor nerves. The faster performing limb would be preferred, its functions more rapidly exercised and its performance more effective. It would also become more practiced than the other as the effects of choice began to operate. It could be argued of course that differential speed of motor nerve conduction is itself a reflection of the superior status of the hemisphere giving rise to it. Nonetheless, such an argument involves greater complexity than one in terms of speed of nerve conduction, and if it were possible to support the latter view then it may be advisable to do so.

Another approach which seems equally capable of explaining the facts but one also which does not rely on the view that one hemisphere exerts exclusive and over-riding control over the other, although this is still possible, is that differences in hand preference or preference for other members of the lateral motor system relate exclusively to the system for motor output and not to the mechanisms for perception or decision. This view has been put forward by Dimond (1970b). If the situation can be envisaged in which two typists are at work in an office and one typist is better than the other. Given a free choice, which one would be chosen to type the decisions of the Board of Governors? The better would be chosen. At the same time, the typist does not make the decisions which she types. She is instrumental in translating decisions made elsewhere. The hands could be regarded in this light. They are the instruments by which the decisions of the brain are expressed. Each is controlled by an effective motor output system. If the motor output system regulating the activities of one hand is more sophisticated relative to that of the other, then not only will it perform better as an instrument, but it will be chosen in preference to the other.

To replicate the effects of handedness the essential element is that the motor output system of one hemisphere should be more proficient than that of the other in order that decisions are channelled through it. Thus we contrast a simple superiority mechanism with the suppression or inhibition view and just as one cannot assume that the secretary is the source of a decision, it may not follow that because the right dominant hand is linked to the left hemisphere, that the latter is exclusively concerned with the processes of decision.

It is difficult to obtain critical evidence, and the problem must await further investigation. However, the view that the differences in the performances of the hands reflect the relative efficiency of the motor output is less complicated. The view of lateral preference as relating to the motor output system is a relatively simple hypothesis for which much data can be advanced in support. It has the advantage of providing a simpler framework for experiment than the suggestion of differences in the perceptual or decision mechanisms.

We may have to accept that the control over the hand by a particular hemisphere may not be as consistent and fixed as we had thought previously. Dimond (1970b) has pointed out that the decision processes of either hemisphere may be expressed through the motor functions of either hand. In the normal intact brain, cross talk takes place over the corpus callosum and the cerebral hemispheres could be considered to be in a state of constant flux. As a consequence, the functions of a particular hand could at one time be governed by the contralateral hemisphere, the one which we have come to imagine as the one to which it belongs, but also the functions of the same hand could be controlled by the other through cross-talk over the corpus callosum. The hand could at one time be controlled by one hemisphere and at another time by the other. In other words the hand need not belong to a hemisphere nor need it be the exclusive province of that one hemisphere to control either the hand or the opposite hemisphere. Knowledge of the function of the corpus callosum makes the fact of the anatomical link between the limb and the contralateral hemisphere appear less important. Control nonetheless has to occur via the output hemisphere. If interchange of control is a marked feature capacities can be expressed through the hand employing them, although such capacities may be localized either in the one or the other hemisphere. For example, a switching arrangement can be envisaged which interconnects language or visuo-spatial functions to either hand in order that the latter may be expressed through the performance of the hand.

Perhaps each hand should no longer be regarded as bearing an exclusive relationship to the contralateral hemisphere. Because the right hand is preferred over the left its hemisphere may not possess an overall mandate for control. Knowledge about the corpus callosum suggests not only that the functions of the contralateral hemisphere are available to the performance of the hand but that the functions of the other hemisphere may be available also. Although the means of higher control may be somewhat fluid, the motor output functions are not so. Most of the differences observed in handedness and lateral motor preference can be attributed to separate and distinct motor output systems on each side, which form the final route for the brain to control the functions of the hand.

VISION

In considering the asymmetries which arise in human function it is as well to bear in mind that handedness, whilst a prominent feature of lateral preference, may be only one of many aspects of right- or left-sidedness. Preferences may be exhibited also in the use of the sense organs.

According to Hildreth (1949) the percentage of the population showing dominance of the right eye varies between 62 and 73 per cent and between 21 and 30 per cent for dominance of the left, the rest show no dominance or dominance which is ambiguous. Groden (1969) more recently studied eye preference in a group of 145 schoolchildren and reported that 53 per cent preferred the use of the right eye, 25 per cent the left and 22 per cent were of undecided preference.

Tests for ocular dominance usually require the subject to perform a task in which only one eye can be used at a time, for example, looking into a microscope or looking through a keyhole or looking through a tube. Tests of this kind indicate that when required to choose one eye rather than the other, consistent patterns of preference emerge but the exact significance of this is difficult to establish. The proportion of people consistently using a particular eye is more nearly balanced than the proportion using a particular hand. Also, the test may be somewhat artificial in that the subject might prefer the use of two eyes rather than one as he is constrained by the situation. That which is accomplished with the use of one eye may often be the equal of that accomplished by the other. It could be misleading to suppose that because one eye is chosen consistently that the other eye is likely to prove itself to be the inferior or necessarily different in capacity. On the contrary the evidence points to the view that the striking feature of a comparison between the eyes is their similarity in function and not their differences.

We have so far considered the function of the eye as a whole. There are differences, however, when we consider the finer detail of visual hemi-field function. Eason et al. (1967) report that the aptitude of evoked responses of the occipital cortex in man differs with stimulation of different visual fields. In the first tests, admittedly using only three left-handed subjects, greater responses occurred when the stimulus appeared in the left visual field. Subsequent tests of a larger number of both right- and left-handed subjects showed that the magnitude of the response of the right lobe relative to that of the left was greater for left-handed subjects. It is not clear what this implies but it does show that visual signals have differential effects depending on which side they stimulate, and this relates to the handedness of the subjects. In other investigations visual evoked responses have been reported not to show asymmetry. Vaughan *et al.* (1964) report that whilst with monocular stimulation a greater response is recorded on the contralateral side, nonetheless, no asymmetry from the right to the left was noted and Gazzaniga (1970) has found no relationship at all of evoked cortical potential to various kinds of perceptual function and is inclined to doubt the tie-up of this measure with other types of hemisphere function.

Laterality effects may be observed on a number of indices. For example, in the use of the Jasper phi-movement test it is recorded that there are cerebral dominance effects in the direction of perceived apparent movement between two stationary light sources when they alternate with one another. Carter (1953) also reports that a relationship exists between handedness and the predominant direction of apparent movement. Efron (1963) also showed that a light flashed in the left visual field of right-handers must precede one flashed in the right visual field in order to be judged verbally as simultaneous. Mirror image results were found for some if not for all of the left-handed subjects. Simple visual stimuli, from the right visual field may evoke the quickest response in right-handers. Speed of function however may provide only one measure of the accomplishments of the hemisphere. The steadily functioning system can perhaps accomplish much over the longer time span on which the most rapidly acting system fails. For this reason if, for no other, it is essential to view hemisphere function in a broader perspective, to acknowledge the importance of time measures, and to use them but not alone . They should be employed in conjunction with other measures.

The capacity of the visual system has been studied by examining the proficiency of each visual hemi-field. Interest has centred recently on the recognition of alphabetic and numerical material.

Mishkin and Forgays (1952) exposed English words tachistoscopically either to the left or to the right of a central fixation point. They found that there was a greater accuracy of recognition for words exposed to the right of fixation. The subjects were bilingual, and when Yiddish words were similarly exposed there was a trend towards greater accuracy for words presented to the left of fixation. The authors interpreted these results to mean that a more effective neural organization is developed in the respective cerebral hemispheres (left for English, right for Yiddish) as the result of the reading processes specific to each language. It is possible that extra cerebral factors such as the left-right direction of scan of the eyes influences the ease with which words in both languages can be read, but this holds only for verbal material.

A number of workers have since reported that the recognition for groups of English letters exposed tachistoscopically on either side of a central fixation point is more accurate when these letters occur to the right of a central fixation point (Orbach, 1953; Forgays, 1953; Harcum and Jones, 1962; Harcum and Finkel, 1963). At the same time the reverse appears to be true for Yiddish words (Orbach, 1953). In the case of Japanese words (Hirata and Osaka, 1967), these are recalled better from the right visual field whether presented unilaterally or bilaterally. The authors state that the written characteristics of Japanese could consistently favour material in the right visual field.

After studies had been conducted which investigated the speed of recognition of material presented to each hemi-field separately, the next task was to present material in both the hemi-fields to see which provides the better recognition. Heron (1957) found, contrary to previous findings, that material presented bilaterally (i.e. on both sides of the fixation point), was recognized considerably better in the left visual field. Heron was led to believe that after the stimulus material had been exposed, a left-right scanning of the rapidly decaying memory trace occurs, leading left visual field to be recalled in preference to that of the right. It is also possible to present a hemispheric view of this situation and to suppose that although the left hemisphere may be the superior in accuracy of recognition of verbal material and although it may function somewhat quicker, nonetheless, the right is more adept at distinguishing one message from the interference caused by another and registers its message more effectively. Even if there are directional scanning effects the problem cannot remain there. The question is how we come to recognize stimulus material in the first place, and how we learn to select some stimuli for response in preference to others. The problem has not been answered, its boundaries have been extended still further.

Kimura (1961) suggested that right field superiority related to left hemisphere functions and Bryden (1964) in reviewing the data from several recognition experiments, supports the view that tachistoscopically presented verbal material is more readily analyzed in the hemisphere in which speech is represented. These effects can be over-ridden, however, by either highly learned or practised acts, such as those employing directional scanning from left to right as occurs in the reading of Hebrew, also through the factors of competitive encounters between the right and the left visual hemi-fields.

In support of this view he showed that single letters and groups of letters may be identified more readily when they appear in the right visual field both when presented in the customary orientation and when their orientation is reversed (Bryden, 1966). He supposed that directional scanning is less important than the hemisphere to which the material is directed. White (1970) is more inclined to attribute the differences which exist in the recognition of groups of letters to memory and learning factors rather than perceptual ones. On a signal detection task in which the subjects were shown half-field displays of four letters exposed for 50 milliseconds and required to decide whether a particular probe letter was present, and to rate the decision on a five point scale, no appreciable differences were reported between one hemi-field and the other. It looked from this experiment as though the differences shown in earlier experiments related to the way in which the coded perceptual material was linked with the memory processes and the mechanisms for articulation. This supported a view of independent capacity of each hemisphere to analyse and code the stimulus material.

Studies of the perception of non-verbal stimuli have been undertaken. Terrace (1959) showed that although superior performance for letters to the left of fixation is a characteristic feature, nonetheless, performance is equal with respect to geometrical forms presented on both sides of fixation, although the subjects had no prior knowledge of which type of material was to appear. Terrace concluded that the direction of the perceptual process was affected by the characteristics of the exposed stimulus. No significant differences between one visual hemi-field and the other in the capacity to recognize geometric figures were found by other authors (Bryden and Rainey, 1963; Heron, 1957) or with regard to nonsense figures (Heron, 1957), although an important distinction here is whether stimulus material is presented in two fields or not. Powell (1962) and Kimura (1963) reported differences in the enumeration of dots. There was a trend for dots to be more accurately reported when they appeared in the left visual field.

Kimura (1966) also reports that enumeration of non-alphabetical stimuli, was more accurate when they appeared in the left visual field. This included nonsense figures as well as groups of dots. Kimura concluded that the left posterior part of the brain plays an important role in the identification of verbal-conceptual forms while the corresponding ones on the right perform other functions in the registration of non-verbal stimuli.

In subsequent studies Kimura (1969) required the subjects to map in a spatial position the location of a single dot shown in either the right or left visual field. Simple detection was found not to be more accurate in one field than another but on localization the males showed left visual field superiority whereas this was absent or reduced in the female group. Kimura points out that visuo-spatial ability could be more differentiated in males than in females.

Asymmetries have been revealed in much of the work carried out by the present author. In some of the first studies (Dimond, 1968, 1970d) it was suggested that there is a special relationship between learning performance and asymmetrical function. If the person had been allowed to practise responses with only the left hand, the addition of a simultaneous right-hand response had little effect. In other words, after practice, left-hand responses were organized such that they proceeded without the possibility of interference affecting them at the stage of organization. With the right hand the situation was different. The addition of a simultaneous left-hand response caused considerable interference with ongoing response. However this is interpreted it is clear that even after practice the responses of the right hand are more sensitive to interference from the addition of a contralateral response than are those of the left. This result held furthermore for both right- and left-handed subjects suggesting that the effects of training operate consistently.

In experiments in which information was projected to separate hemispheres asymmetries of function were again found. it should be pointed out first however that in simple response situations no differences were observed between the performance of one hand and the other (Dimond, 1969a, 1970c), neither were differences observed in simple response times when information was projected to one hemisphere rather than another (Dimond, 1970c). However, when two signals were projected to each hemisphere simultaneously, each demanding response from the hands, a certain degree of response blocking was observed as has been stated previously. However, blocking was less pronounced when signals were projected to the single left hemisphere than when they were directed to the right hemisphere. Such a result is consonant with the view of more rapid organization of motor functions by the left hemisphere. In a further experiment (Dimond, 1969a) it is reported that the asymmetries observed in response blocking hold not only for signals directed simultaneously to the one hemisphere, either the right or the left, but also in respect of signals arriving one a short period after the other. In other words there are differences in the degree of refractoriness between one hemisphere and the other. Response to the second signal is delayed if both the first and the second signal are projected to the same hemisphere. The delay in response to the second signal is marked when both are directed to the left hemisphere, but it is extended considerably over and above this when both signals are projected to the right hemisphere (Dimond, 1969a).

Similar considerations apply when language material is employed in place of visual stimuli for reaction time responses. In a further experiment Dimond (1971a) showed that two sequences of letters each forming a four-letter word when projected together simultaneously to either the right or the left hemisphere, are registered more successfully when directed to the left than to the right.

This again illustrates asymmetry of function. However, caution has to be exercised to dispel the belief that the asymmetry is a totally one-sided affair. In the same investigation (Dimond, 1971a) it was shown that if one sequence of letters is projected to one hemisphere at the same time as another sequence is projected to the other hemisphere, as an alternative to the projection of both sequences to the same hemisphere, then the message directed to the right hemisphere is registered in preference to that directed to the left. This could not be explained by left to right scanning because left/right visual field differences were not observed when the material was projected to the single hemisphere. This suggests that although the left hemisphere may have the greater capacity for dealing with large quantities of concurrent information, nonetheless, for reasons which we cannot as yet specify, there are qualities of function which ensure that when given a choice the right wins out and registers its information more effectively than the other. This result cautions against the premature dismissal of the right as insignificant and inferior in its function to the left.

We now have the task of considering exactly how these results from the study of the visual processes relate to what we know of brain function. It is possible to regard differences between one side and the other as a straightforward manifestation of the differences between the cerebral hemispheres in their functions. Kimura (1966) supposes that the left posterior part of the brain contributes critically to the identification of verbal conceptual forms, but at the same time she states that there is no good evidence that it is of crucial importance for the perception of other kinds of visual stimuli. In fact, she suggests that her data support the view that the corresponding region of the right hemisphere is predominant for some process as yet ill-defined, involved in the enumeration of nonverbal stimuli. Certainly the results would support the view that there are differences in the processes of visual perception between one hemisphere and the other. The left hemisphere (in a right-handed population) showing a superiority in the speed and accuracy of recognition or even perhaps the capacity to report on written language forms, and the other hemisphere showing evidence of some superiority in respect of non-language aspects of visual perception. However, we may not want to emphasize that the recognition of language and non-language forms have nothing in common.

At the same time as acknowledging that asymmetries in visual function exist, there are some contradictions in the literature which lead one to suppose that these asymmetries may not be as definite as other authors suppose. The temptation also must be avoided of supposing that because a superiority can be demonstrated for one side that the other takes no part whatsoever in organization. In the case of ocular dominance it is possible to use only one eye at a time in many of the tests. The fact that one eye is consistently chosen and preferred over the other does not mean that the other functions any less as an eye. Similarly, with regard to the differences between one visual field and another, the visual field recognizing verbal material best does not do so to the total exclusion of any recognition in the other half field. Material is recognized and reported in both visual half-fields, but one shows superiority. The results themselves do not support an all or none interpretation.

Taking into account that each visual hemi-field has considerable capacity for recognition of material of all types, and that the asymmetries which exist form a relatively small part of the variance over and above this, it is possible to ask whether the difference could be attributed to the sense organs themselves. It is a difficult hypothesis to rule out but it seems most likely, all things considered, that the major differences do not occur here but are to be found in the functions of the cerebral hemispheres. The functions of either side appear on the whole to be somewhat similar, but biases operate over and above the similarities. It cannot be assumed that the biases all go one way and that of necessity one hemisphere predominates over the other all the time, because the nature of the bias depends at least to some extent on the stimulus material used. In some cases the right may prove to be the superior, and in other cases the left. Ignoring the fact for the moment that biases operate and that one side may be somewhat superior to the other, potential apparently exists for the registration of material on either side. If the equation is made between visual hemifield and cerebral hemisphere, the fact emerges that information projected to either hemisphere is registered well and accurately in most instances. Leaving aside the bias this would argue that each hemisphere acting as a receptive system has capacity for the registration of information, and that to a large extent the hemispheres duplicate the capacities of one other in information receiving functions. If we were to adopt the simplest argument and relate the material transmitted through each visual half-field as being a direct measure of the function of the hemisphere to which it is projected, the picture we would obtain would be one in which each had considerable capacity for the registration of information not all that different from the other, although biases towards one or the other would still be seen. At the same time complex interactions could take place between the one and the other after the information has first been registered and subsequently analysed. It should not be assumed that because a predominance occurs that this necessarily implies that the cerebral hemisphere exercises control to the total exclusion of the other over that function. It seems more likely that in the intact brain there is an interplay between one and the other in the ultimate translation of analysed and coded information into action.

AUDITORY FUNCTIONS

Differences are also to be observed between performance on one ear and that on the other. Kimura (1961a) presented two sets of digits simultaneously to both ears, and showed that those presented to the right are recalled more successfully than those presented to the left ear. In other words there is superiority for the right ear and it is tempting to speculate that this implies superiority for the corresponding left hemisphere specific to this task.

Damage to the left temporal lobe impaired performance irrespective of the ear to which the stimuli were presented (Kimura, 1961a), and temporal lobectomy on either side impaired recognition at the ear contralateral to the removal. Kimura (1961b) also reports that in patients with epileptogenic foci in various parts of the brain, for those with speech represented in the left hemisphere the right ear was more efficient for verbal recall and for those with speech represented in the right hemisphere the left ear was more efficient, this effect proved itself to be independent of handedness. Oxbury and Oxbury (1969) support Kimura's findings that left temporal lobectomy was followed by an impaired ability to report digits presented to the right ear. However, the ability to report digits presented to the left ear was unaltered. The impairment was most marked following excisions which included the whole of the transverse gyri of Heschl.

Subjects respond faster to right ear stimulation on reaction time tasks when they do not know which ear is to be stimulated. Also they were faster on binaural than monaural trials, but when they knew in advance which ear was to be stimulated the previous differences were no longer apparent (Simon, 1967). Although Bakker (1969) has reported that there may be ear asymmetry effects with monaural stimulation when a prescribed order of recall is forced upon the subject. Generally this superiority of the right ear occurs only when competition operates between one ear and the other. Under monaural conditions these differences do not form a noteworthy feature of the results (Kimura, 1963, 1964; Palmer, 1964).

It should not be assumed on the basis of these results that superiority in dichotic stimulation experiments is unequivocably and invariably displayed by the right ear. The predominance achieved by the ear depends on the type of material and when non-verbal stimuli are used, superiority may be displayed by the left and not the right ear (Milner, 1962). Kimura (1964) reported that melodies are perceived with greater efficiency by the left ear, and she attributes right ear superiority to the predominance of the left hemisphere for speech, and the left ear superiority to the specialization of the right hemisphere for non-verbal functions such as music. Kimura (1967) also, in a paper reviewing the evidence relating to lateral asymmetry, again points to the left ear as the superior in melodic pattern recognition. Kimura and Folb (1968) reported that when sounds such as those produced by reverse playback of recorded speech were presented to the right and the left ears, the sounds arriving at the right ear were more accurately identified than those arriving at the left. These findings are comparable with those for normal speech sounds.

Kimura (1970) has reported that certain sounds presented in the dichotic situation are heard better through the left than the right ear. Speech also when chopped into segments of 200 milliseconds or less no longer produces a superior response on the right ear, but instead shows the superior response in the left. Kimura suggests that in sections of this brevity speech is no longer registered as such and remains undifferentiated by the brain from other types of noise. These results demonstrate that the right ear is not the superior on all tests of function, and if an equation is made between the ear and the contralateral hemisphere they suggest that the right hemisphere can be the superior on certain tasks.

In this connection Shankweiler (1966) studied patients with temporal lobe lesions on dichotic listening tests, one consisting of melodies and the other of digits. Perception of dichotically presented melodies was selectively impaired by right temporal lobectomy, whereas perception of dichotically presented digits was selectively impaired by left temporal lobectomy.

It was not long before tests of this kind became incorporated as an experimental method in child psychology.

The right ear effect operates as early as the age of four (Kimura, 1963b). However, the boys showed a lower total score than the girls at the early ages, and the results suggest that boys lag behind girls in the capacity to perceive speech. Sinclair (1968) in another study, reports that the effect may be established as early as the third year of life. Bakker (1967) on the other hand, could find no evidence of the superiority of the right ear for the recall of digits in 5-12 year old children, but he did find that morse-like sound patterns were better retained when presented to the left ear and presumably this reflects the underlying rhythmic pattern and time distributed sequence of melodic line on other tests.

Knox and Kimura (1970) found in their study of children between the ages of five and eight, that more non-verbal sounds were correctly identified from the left than the right ear, whereas verbal material produced a right ear superiority. Kimura suggests that the asymmetry for non-verbal sounds exists by at least the age of five. Boys showed themselves to be better at registering non-verbal sounds than girls. The development of asymmetry for verbal material, and for other types of stimulus, has a definite onset early in childhood.

Many further studies have been undertaken to specify what factors lead to the greatest effect. Delay between stimuli has been shown to be important. In right-handed undergraduates a very strong right ear preference was obtained with delays of right channel information as great as 30 milliseconds (Mehlman, 1969). Shock also may have differential effects. Murphy and Venables (1969) in their study showed that the performance of the right and the left ear does not differ when clicks are presented alone. However, the presentation of a short electric shock before a click is due results in a considerable decrement in right ear performance but little change in left ear performance. Murphy and Venables suggest that the hemispheres may differ in their lability or in cortico-reticular interactions and the results are in line with the investigations of the interfering effects of an additional response on a previously operating response of the hands (Dimond, 1970d). Shock, as measured by G S R can be suppressed more effectively by ongoing verbal activity if this occurs in the right as opposed to the left ear (Bever et al., 1968). The response to shock is less during the beginning of a clause than at its end, but this effect is magnified to speech presented through the right ear.

Some criticism has been made of the view that the difference between the ears in auditory perception necessarily represents better perception of material presented to the right ear than that presented to the left. Inglis (1965) has suggested that differences in the capacity for immediate memory may explain the reported effect.

The view that the difference between one ear and the other is necessarily one of perception has also been criticized by Oxbury et al. (1967). They point out that the order of report is likely to have a significant effect upon the accuracy with which the information from both sides is recalled. In their investigation in which they randomized the order of report, there are no significant differences between performance on the right ear and that on the left. There was, however, a difference between the first channel to be reported and the second. They suggest that an attentional bias towards the right ear may explain the superiority when free recall is allowed.

In a vigorous defence of the earlier interpretation, Satz (1968) points out that when the order of report is controlled as it has been in a number of experiments, then the right ear may still show itself to be the superior.

There are reports in the literature where investigators have failed to show the desired effect. This may be because they have used particular methods which do not allow the effect to emerge clearly. Some of the inconsistency could be explained by the suggestion that the effect is revealed by some procedures more than others.

Brunt and Goetzinger (1968) found for example when the same subjects were tested, that the results indicated a significant right ear dominance effect for the Kimura and Katz tests but not for the Dirks test. Clearly the results depend at least to some degree on the type of test used. Despite these difficulties there exists a substantial body of evidence for the effects. Before it is concluded that various specializations operate in the brain for different types of material however there are several further points to be considered.

The differences in response as the result of presenting the message through one ear or the other in the dichotic situation, although significant are still in fact slight. It is not the case that one sense organ receives the message totally at the expense of the other. Broadbent and Gregory (1964) state that whilst the results would not perhaps by themselves be very convincing evidence of a priority for the right ear, they are sufficient to confirm the difference already established by Bryden and Kimura. Secondly, it must be remembered that although a superiority may be established for one ear, there is still a considerable capacity for function through the other ear. Thirdly, the effect does not generally appear under conditions of mon-aural stimulation, but only when messages find themselves in competition with one another.

It is possible that the bias which comes about does so through the selectivity of mechanisms at the ears themselves. It is not the intention to suggest that the ear carries out the complex processes necessary to the analysis of a verbal message or a melodic line, but simply that it has a differential attenuation. This seems unlikely however because of the difficulty of distinguishing for example between music and speech which are both characterized by intonation, rhythm, and sequential line. It could not even be argued that timbre could allow a distinction because melodies can be sung as well as played. We have therefore to resort to an explanation involving the functions of the cerebral hemispheres themselves.

If the right ear indicates left hemisphere function and vice versa with verbal material we see a situation in which the left hemisphere emerged the superior, but the right came a close second. Because one side shows a superiority, it has often been ,supposed that the same side has exclusive exercise over the function but at the same time the other side may have a capacity for that function as well, and the capacity of the hemisphere coming second should be given some recognition.

There is often a tendency presumably because language has been studied at the expense of other functions to regard laterality effects as indicating a one-sidedness of brain function. Here again caution is necessary because whilst one hemisphere appears to predominate in language functions, the other exceeds in perception of sound patterns and melodic line as well as in the perception of spatial events.

The results indicate that no one hemisphere is totally predominant and that there are residuals in the secondary ear which suggest largely unrecognized abilities for the exercise of particular functions.

CONCLUSIONS

There is some foreshadowing of asymmetrical function in the brain of primates closely related to man, but this tends to take the form of preference for the use of one limb rather than another. Taking the picture as a whole, most animals are ambilateral, and the numbers preferring one limb are closely matched by those preferring the other.

When the human brain is considered, asymmetries are demonstrated at a variety of levels which include motor functions and perception. It could be supposed that these asymmetries are characteristic and that they differentiate man from non-human animals. The question arises as to what significance attaches to asymmetry. Some authors suppose that the brain is more or less totally asymmetrical in function, and that it is dominated in control exclusively by one side. This seems to be an exaggerated view. Certainly it is possibe to over-emphasize asymmetry at the expense of the functional similarity which exists between one hemisphere and the other.

If the brain of man is totally different from the brain of animals then asymmetry may be taken as one example of its special properties. If, on the other hand, there is an evolutionary ontinuum and man is an advanced but nonetheless representative member, the basic similarities can be stressed and the human brain regarded as conforming to the same bilaterally symmetrical design, but that imposed over and above this design are certain asymmetries which have been previously described.

When the subject is faced with a choice between systems, one or other lateral system may emerge the superior. In this chapter we have asked if this implies a brain organization in which one side has an exclusive exercise over function. The fact of priority signifies that a relationship exists between the two, but at the same time reflects only a small area of this relationship, too small to base an argument which denies capacities to the other. Care should be taken that such over-generalization is not made about hemisphere function.

It could be supposed that the left is superior in most important respects and therefore the dominant or controlling hemisphere. But much of this superiority rests in a specialization for language which we shall discuss later, while the right possesses its own specialities too. A view which supposes that the left is always dominant does not do justice to the evidence of tasks in which the right emerges the superior.

The facts need to be considered. But is it possible that these facts themselves are of somewhat limited significance when the problem of control is discussed? For example, in the case of a businessman and his secretary, the secretary receives messages and replies to letters. The decisions rest with the businessman, yet superficially the secretary appears to do all the work. No one is suggesting that the right hemisphere rather than the left is the controller of the brain as a whole. The analogy is used merely to suggest that the problem of control is a very complicated one, and that the methods available to us at present may only go some way towards determining the nature of the chain of command. If we studied messages passing to and from the office, we might conclude that control rested exclusively with the secretary, and we might imagine the businessman to be redundant because we have no knowledge of the way in which he transmits his decisions to the secretary. Certainly, on the basis of present-day asymmetry studies, it is impossible to single out either hemisphere as the controller because not all functions are associated with one hemisphere alone, and so far we only know about those associations which we have been fortunate enough to study. Although frequently interpreted as favouring one hemisphere more than the other in the exercise of a particular function, the evidence might just as easily be interpreted as favouring an association between hemispheres because of the statistical structure of the results. It seems highly probable that capacities are distributed on both sides of the brain and that the cross-talk is instrumental in coordinating activities between them.

8

Language

p89→76

INTRODUCTION

An obvious relationship between speech and the functions of the left hemisphere has been demonstrated from early times in the history of human neurological investigation. It is not our intention to question ~~what seems to be one of the best attested facts in the literature~~ However, in discussing the cortical localization of the language processes, it is necessary to differentiate between speech itself as output in an articulated form, and linguistic processes which form the antecedent links in the chain of the language process and which ultimately lead to speech output. What may be true of the final events in this system may not be necessarily true of prior events, however closely each are related. The person who is deaf and dumb and has never acquired the capacity to speak may be able to communicate in other ways. The person suffering from aphasia after surgery may also have preserved the capacity to communicate in other ways. It is possible to lose the capacity for speech, for example after operation on the brain, and yet show no impairment in what might be called higher linguistic functions.

Siger (1968) makes the point in his article *Gestures the language of signs and communication,* that extensive non-verbal communication is a feature of normal behaviour and that there is a long history of linguistic processes being expressed through artificial languages like that employed by the deaf. Language of this kind, whilst perhaps lacking the sophistication of speech, possesses both a sequence, a grammar and a syntax. The cortical mechanisms involved are as yet little understood.

In normal right-handed individuals speech and language mechansisms are represented in the cortex of the left hemisphere. Speech disturbances of a greater or lesser kind occur in cases of apoplexy in which there is a hemiplegia of the right side of the body, whereas in patients whose strokes produce a left hemiplegia, disturbance of speech is uncommon. In cases of cerebral tumour, abscesses, aneurysms and acute open head injuries, the same rule holds. Although speech and language functions in the adult are undoubtedly lateralized to the left hemisphere, there is evidence that equipotentiality occurs during the

162

very early years. There is also evidence that the right hemisphere as well as subcortical mechanisms may be implicated in the production of language.

PARALANGUAGE

The reasons for specifying animal communication as language are not hard to find. Language follows a sequential pattern and it is not difficult to detect serial ordering in most animal communications whether vocal or non-vocal. Language follows certain rules and the notion of syntax is something which also finds its place in the study of animal communication. Busnel (1968) argues that if the signal as such has a recognizable temporal structure and thus a composite one, its structure is syntactic. Thirdly, language has meaning. The question of meaning in communication produced considerable confusion. Meaning surely implies a change of state. A message can be said to have been delivered if a change of state is induced in the receiver. Meaning in this sense is certainly characteristic of animal communication.

On these and other grounds we can describe animal communication as paralanguage—a system possessing many features in common with true language.

Much non-verbal behaviour of human beings also takes the form of paralanguage. It has sequential order and it too is susceptible to analysis in terms of a formal grammar. There seems no a priori reason to attribute grammatical statement only to speech functions. Lashley (1951) argued that not only speech but all skilled acts seem to involve the same problems of serial ordering, even down to the temporal coordination of muscular contractions in movements, for example those of reaching and grasping. Lashley went on to argue that the nervous mechanisms underlying order in the more primitive acts may contribute ultimately to the solution even of the physiology of logic.

Stimulation of the premotor area seldom gives rise to impulses passing to isolated muscles but causes the development of complex motor synergies involving whole motor systems (Fritsch and Hitzig, 1870; Penfield, 1950). Lesion of the premotor area leads to disturbance of integrated muscle movements in the monkey and lesion of the premotor area of man has similar effects. Movements become clumsy and their individual components are no longer combined into integrated motor systems. Luria (1966) stated that the role of the premotor cortex in the organization of human behaviour has been imperfectly investigated and only isolated accounts of patients with lesions of the premotor system are to be found in the literature. The case Luria describes suffered a bilateral premotor lesion in the midline. He showed as a principal defect an inability in the ordering of motor sequences. The patient said when asked to perform tasks such as opening and closing the fist of each hand in sequence, 'Something is holding my hand back, it will not work properly'. Similar difficulties were observed in tapping out rhythms.

The difficulties of this patient were not confined to this. Within a day or two after being wounded he noticed difficulty in his speech which was no longer fluent but impeded and fragmentary. The patient reported that if he wants to say something then the words stick and he can say nothing. The disturbance of speech persisted as a permanent feature of the syndrome.

Luria points out that both in the study of the patients skilled movements and in the study of his speech processes a basic disturbance was found in the scheme for the sequencing of events, a disturbance of activity consisting of a series of consecutive actions, or what Luria described as the higher automatisms.

Several features of this work are important. One is that there are lesions which disturb not the operation of simple movements, but the complex sequencing of movements and the integration of movements into chains. If the capacity to coordinate and integrate sequences of behaviour represents the basic mechanisms by which paralanguage in a human being is controlled, then we can go some way towards establishing a site for the control of functions of this kind.

The second point is that the disorder of the sequencing of movements is something occurring not only in skilled motor performance but also in speech. Articulation, is after all, the expression of a sequence of movements and the results suggest that there may be some common factor in the mechanism for the control of body movement, and that for control of the speech processes.

LANGUAGE AND THE LEFT HEMISPHERE

The history of the study of aphasia has been reviewed by a number of authors (Critchley, 1961, 1970; Joynt, 1964; Benton, 1964b). It is possible only to refer to this history briefly here. Dax has been proposed as the forerunner of the study of the cerebral localization of the speech processes. It seems likely that the major stimulus to such investigations came from the work of Broca (1865) who reported that a lesion of an area of association cortex lying anterior to the lower end of the left motor cortex disrupts the capacity for articulated speech. Mutism is, however, rare in these cases and some capacity to issue words remains. The speech is often described as telegraphic and there may be a comparable writing difficulty. When, however, the understanding of spoken or written language is considered there may be little, if any, impairment. Geschwind (1970) regards this type of lesion as commonly disrupting established movement patterns of the speech organs. There may be a severe accompanying paralysis of the arm or the leg, in most cases more severe in respect of the arm. Speech disorder is usually gross in the right-handed person if the lesion occurs in the left hemisphere. The followers of Broca expressed the view that a special relationship existed between speech functions and the left hemisphere.

Bastian (1869) and Schmidt (1871) described cases of aphasia in which not only speech but comprehension was impaired. Wernicke (1874, 1906) also described such cases and extended the typology of aphasia in pointing to sensory varieties. Post-mortem material showed a different localization from that described by Broca. Wernicke singled out the cortex of the posterior superior temporal region as of importance. Central aphasia or conduction aphasia has been described by Goldstein (1948). This is regarded as arising from a lesion of the arcuate fasciculus, a region connecting Wernicke's area to Broca's area. The patient has a fluent aphasia in which errors of speech are common, the patient often failing to find the correct word.

Geschwind (1967) shows also that a large lesion running through the parietal region effectively cuts off connections running to and from Wernicke's area. Fluent aphasia is produced and in this case comprehension may also be impaired. There is substantial evidence that speech disorders of the type described relate predominantly to lesion of the left hemisphere.

In their studies of the electrical stimulation of the cortex Penfield and Roberts (1959) did not completely uphold the view of rigidly defined anatomical speech areas. However, they were able to obtain responses from regions regarded as the classical speech areas but also from a third area in the supplementary motor area anterior to that controlling the movements of the foot. Evidence for the role of this additional area has also been produced in the studies of Russell and Young (1969).

With the introduction of the intracarotid sodium amytal test by Wada (1949) it became possible to compare the two cerebral hemispheres for the first time in a single patient for speech output. Some of the most extensive observations in its use are those of Branch et al. (1964) who tested 123 patients and required them to name objects and to count following injection. The majority of right-handed patients had speech on the left side. When clinical evidence was found of an injury to the left hemisphere at birth or in early life speech was found to be on the right side in approximately two-thirds of the left-handed patients.

When no clinical evidence existed of early left-sided brain damage, speech was found to be on the left in two-thirds of the left-handed and ambidextrous patients.

Approximately one-tenth of the right-handed patients had speech on the right side of the brain and in none of these patients was there bilateral representation but in some of the left-handed and ambidextrous patients there was.

Evidence for the relationship of language disorder to the side of lesion has been reviewed by Piercy (1964) and Zangwill (1963, 1964). Ettlinger et al. (1955) were able to trace in the literature only 15 cases of dysphasia resulting from right hemisphere lesions in right-handed persons. Espir and Russell (1961) and Penfield and Roberts (1959) suggested that the incidence of dysphasia is probably about 1 per cent or slightly more when the lesion is right-sided, and about 67 per cent when the lesion is left-sided. Zangwill (1960) in his analysis of the literature relates aphasia to handedness and suggests that there is strong evidence that among people who are generally regarded as left-handed dysphasia more often than not results from a left than from a right hemisphere lesion. Blakemore and Falconer (1967) and Milner (1962) all show that patients with left hemisphere temporal lobectomy show a marked impairment of verbal behaviour and Newcombe (1969) points out that men with left hemisphere lesions show a residual but consistent deficit which was not, however invariably related to a clinically detectable dysphasia but was nonetheless a prominent feature of the results. Patients with left hemisphere lesions are not only deficient in word fluency tasks but also in the primary registration and in the learning of verbal material. The clinical evidence therefore is overwhelming of the association of lesions of the left hemisphere with disturbances of language and the articulation of speech.

EARLY SPEECH DEVELOPMENT AND EQUIPOTENTIALITY

The language functions of young children have received attention over the past few years because of the relevance to an understanding of speech pathology and to an understanding of the relationships of speech function to brain mechanisms.

The cerebral hemispheres appear to be equipotential in respect of language involvement during the early years. Lenneberg (1967) quotes evidence to show that if after the age of the acquisition of language (between 20-36 months of age) the child is affected by cerebral trauma then whatever beginning had been made with speech development appears to be lost and the stages of the acquisition of language have to be passed through again. However, cerebral trauma to either hemisphere appears at this age to have equal and opposite effects.

Basser (1962) states that there is a period during infancy at which the hemispheres are equipotential. In approximately half the children with brain lesions sustained during the first two years of life the onset of speech is delayed, the rest, however, begin to speak at the normal time.

This distribution is the same irrespective of the side of the lesion, i.e. children with left hemisphere lesions show delayed onset of speech as frequently as those with right hemisphere lesions. Data from Basser (1962).

	Onset of Speech		
	Normal	Delayed	Never
Left Hemisphere	18	15	1
Right Hemisphere	19	15	4

Basser (1962) takes this to indicate that during the first two years of life cerebral dominance is not yet well established. Boone (1965) also reports that a severe and persistent aphasia rarely occurred from unilateral cerebral damage of any type before the age of nine or ten years. From that time on there is, however, a greater preponderance of children with left-sided lesions who develop aphasia. Children under nine with aphasia show a remarkably rapid recovery. Sugar (1952) also stated that in children between the age of five and ten years of age, injury to the left hemisphere produced only a temporary aphasia, but after that age language symptoms persist. Evidence from studies of hemispherectomy discussed previously shows that if the child suffers a lesion in early infancy irrespective of side, then the healthy hemisphere eventually takes up the speech function (Basser, 1962).

It is possible that different processes operate when the child is learning about the language than when he is learning to use and to manipulate language. As the child grows older speech disturbances become manifest more often in association with left than with right hemisphere lesions. Basser (1962) quotes evidence that by the time the child has matured sufficiently to have attained speech but has still not reached the age of ten years left-sided lesions result in speech disturbances in 85 per cent of the cases whereas right-sided lesions result in speech disturbances in 45 per cent of the cases. A marked change in laterality occurs during development, but at the same time it should be pointed out that almost half the right-sided lesion group showed speech disturbance, and it must be supposed on this evidence not only that there is an association of speech disturbance with lesions of the left hemisphere, but also that there is at this period an association of speech disturbance with lesions of the right hemisphere.

Penfield (1965) regards the area of cortex which is to be later taken up with language as the uncommitted cortex. As the area is employed for speech it becomes the major speech area or speech cortex. There is some danger of circularity in this argument because the question arises that if the cortex is uncommitted how is it that it becomes used initially for speech. However, the concept of the uncommitted cortex does point to some equipotentiality for development in the early years. Equipotentiality for speech is of great interest. It features during the acquisition of language and lateral differentiation occurs only after language has been acquired. It is commonly supposed that 'dominance for speech' enters in and that somehow this facilitates the complex development of speech. The evidence suggests, however, that lateralization of the speech processes follows only after language acquisition has occurred as the result in so far as we can judge of intense bilateral activity of the brain. Equipotentiality is not simply a statement of the potential for possible language development at a later stage, it is a concept which suggests active involvement and bilateral function at the most intense and earliest periods of the foundation of language. When the magnitude of the task and the speed of language acquisition are considered it is not surprising that the linguistic capacities of each hemisphere appear to be utilized to the full.

At the stage at which the child is learning about language, the cerebral hemispheres show equipotentiality, at a later stage the child is learning to use language and it is at this time we witness the lateralization of the speech processes. Here again we need to make a distinction between speech and linguistic capacity because in the early equipotential stages the linguistic capacities of each hemisphere are employed but it is only later that speech as the output system becomes localized in the left hemisphere. The development of a unilateral system for control of speech need not rob the other hemisphere of the linguistic capacities it apparently demonstrated so ably at an earlier time.

The data of the effects of cerebral trauma occurring before the age of ten years suggest that the left hemisphere develops control of speech output, but that prior to that time both contribute in differing degrees to linguistic function until quite a late age. Equipotentiality in infancy is not only a fact of importance in the acquisition of language, it means also that there is continuity between man and the infra-human species in bilateral organization of the brain at least during the first years of infancy.

LANGUAGE AND THE RIGHT HEMISPHERE

A thorough evaluation of the literature on speech and language disorders presents a formidable task. Reports of case histories vary widely in their accuracy. Some symptoms may be exaggerated at the expense of others, and there are problems in assessing how strongly a particular symptom is represented in each individual case. Lesions can have more than one effect. They may not be an inert but an active site for interference with other more distant mechanisms. Another problem is the varying character of the speech disorders according to whether the patients are in an acute stage of the illness or on the other hand if they have settled into a stable condition. In view of these difficulties the picture which emerges from the study of neurological case material must be a qualified one.

Broca coined the phrase, 'On parle avec l'hémisphère gauche'. This has commonly been taken to mean that speech at all events in its expressive aspect is exclusively controlled with certain exceptions by the left cerebral hemisphere. Zangwill (1967) points out, however, that not all neurologists have held so simple minded a view and he quotes the case of Hughlings Jackson (1874) who held that some speech processes are represented in both hemispheres, and that it is the more highly voluntary and propositional aspects of speech that suffer in aphasia.

It can happen that the speech output system is displaced from its customary position in the left to one in the right hemisphere if certain types of disturbance are present such as a focal epilepsy. Landsell (1962) describes cases in which the speech output system was located by means of the amytal test. The data from these cases show that when the right hemisphere becomes involved in the control of speech output then it also becomes somewhat more involved with the verbal factor as measured by intelligence tests. As regards verbal intelligence it is better for speech to move to the right than to remain in the damaged left hemisphere. This can be explained by the interference to verbal output from an epileptic focus lying in close proximity to the mechanism for speech. Hécaen (1959) expressed a somewhat similar view. In his concept of equipotentiality he implied that either hemisphere can assume the functions of the other although at a reduced level. The potential of one hemisphere for speech although having a distinct and separate existence may not be used except in the case of damage to the other.

The evidence from studies of brain-bisection quoted in a previous chapter supports the view that speech functions show a clear relationship with the left hemisphere but at the same time they suggest that this is largely a specialization for speech output. Nominated objects can certainly be retrieved by touch with the left hand indicating a measure of right hemisphere comprehension. Butler and Norrsell (1968) also found that their patient, a 15-year-old boy, had the capacity to retrieve by touch objects named in either visual half field. Words in the right visual field were vocalized at once, there is no doubt about the right visual field superiority, but the images displayed to the left visual field were sometimes named as well, admittedly after long exposures. Butler and Norrsell suggest that the right hemisphere can demonstrate some undoubted linguistic capacity when the speech mechanisms are captured, in spite of corpus callosum section.

One of the significant findings in relation to the organization of language in normal subjects is that by Schafer (1967). Reliable non-random changes in the electrical activity of the brain designated 'cortical command potentials' have been demonstrated to precede voluntary hand and foot movements, finger pressing, and speech (Ertl and Schafer, 1967).

Average command potentials from the human scalp preceding speech onset are characteristically different for the spoken letters 'T', 'O' and 'P'. This prevails over the left temporal speech area and it confirms what is already known about the relationship of speech functions to this area of the brain. There is also evidence that an area over the right sensori-motor region also produces this cortical activity preceding speech, and in so far as it is possible to specify that this activity represents something of the antecedent links in the chain generating speech, it would seem to relate not only to the left but also to the right cerebral hemisphere.

Previous work using subdural electrodes suggests that command potentials preceding voluntary movements are of cortical origin. Schafer (1967) whilst regarding speculation as to the significance of these potentials as premature does nonetheless suggest that some components at least may be regarded as electrophysiological signs associated with the act of selecting and deciding to speak a given word. This is in accordance with the view that whilst the normal subject may use the left hemisphere to control the output system of speech, antecedent links in the chain leading to speech production are probably present in both hemispheres.

Newcombe, Oldfield and Wingfield (1965) reported that patients with mild nominal aphasia showed differences from the normal population only when the names of objects were chosen whose use occurs less than approximately one per 100,000 words as measured by a standard word count. Oldfield (1966) also supports a view of aphasia as an extension of normal linguistic difficulties. He presents data on brain injured and control subjects in which the latency to name an object is used as an index of retrieval time. Latency measurements were found to discriminate between normals and controls, and seemed to be useful in the study of aphasic disorders. The aphasics came out worse with the highest mean latency. Oldfield reports, however that contrary to the accepted clinical picture the right hemisphere group without aphasia showed itself to be inferior in naming to the left hemisphere group without aphasia. These results suggest that the right hemisphere could play some part in the organization of speech and they could reflect an interrelationship between the hemispheres in the production of language.

Oldfield himself, however, attributes the naming-latency difficulties of the right hemisphere patients to perceptual disorders. Taking only those patients who name all the objects in the series it was found that the latency-frequency curves for right and left hemisphere cases were virtually identical (Newcombe et al., 1971).

Early studies of the association of the language mechanisms with the right or so-called minor hemisphere have been reviewed by Weinstein (1964). Weinstein and Keller (1963) had reported earlier that there are difficulties associated with naming objects which stem from lesions on both sides of the brain. The difficulties are different on the two sides. They suggest that left hemisphere lesions lead to problems with phonetic and semantic categories, but the patient with a right hemisphere lesion does not simply have a mild aphasia but a change in his relationship with the environment. Patients with right hemisphere lesions showing this disorder were all disoriented in respect of place or date and this was expressed through misnaming of the hospital as well as stating an incorrect month of the year and contracting the distance between their own home and the hospital. Weinstein (1964) points out that it is possible to consider other disturbances commonly associated with right hemisphere lesions as a form of language disturbance. Such disturbances have frequently been regarded in the past as disturbances of perception or body image, but they can also relate to the way the person talks about his perceptions or describes his body image.

The question of right hemisphere participation is by no means an open and shut case. Patients with damage to the right hemisphere often display verbal impairment which is, however, not 'aphasic' in nature. In one case described by Taylor (1965) deficiencies in time orientation, copying and writing were disproportionately disturbed and this suggested to Taylor signs of an organic mental syndrome rather than aphasia. At the same time Taylor acknowledged that there are difficulties represented in the linguistic sphere. Marcie et al. (1965) also in a further study of right-handed patients with right hemisphere lesions report that difficulties with respect to speech are experienced which they are inclined to attribute not to disorders of comprehension, but to perseveration; 'le phénomène pe'. This would not appear to be the only explanation, however, because about 50 per cent of the right hemisphere patients showed some difficulty in generating grammatically correct phrases beyond three or four words in length, as well as difficulties in the execution of the more symbolic aspects of reading and writing.

Glonig *et al.* (1969) report observations on 114 patients in which the site of the lesion was verified at autopsy. Aphasic disturbances were observed in patients with both left and right hemisphere lesions, and the findings in this recent study do not support the view that language disturbances are to be observed exclusively in cases of left hemisphere lesion.

The contribution of right hemisphere function has been remarked upon by a number of authors in recent years. The aim has not been to replace localization at the left with that at the right, but to suggest that the right hemisphere plays some role although perhaps a diminished one in the regulation of the speech processes. Eisenson (1962), for example, shows that intellectual language deficits may be assocated with right as well as left hemisphere lesions and he points out the importance of the right cercbral hemisphere in language formulation. Critchley (1962) also expressed the view that the right hemisphere has a contribution to make in the organization of speech. He conceived of speech as a spectrum ranging from the normal subject at one end through to the linguistic pattern of the left (right-handed) full-fledged aphasic patient at the other end. At a half-way station between these two occur the less intense but significant linguistic difficulties of the patient with right hemisphere lesions.

The left hemisphere makes its obvious contribution to speech and language, the right hemisphere contributes also. Now we have to assess something of the interrelation between them in the genesis of language. Before doing that, however, we have to discuss yet another complicating factor and that is the implication of subcortical systems in the control of speech.

HEMISPHERE INTEGRATION AND LANGUAGE

It is not sufficient to regard the speech processes as regulated exclusively by a small area on the surface of the cortex. There is substantial evidence of subcortical involvement, for example, in the attempted surgical alleviation of Parkinsonism in which small lesions are produced by stereotactic techniques, the site selected by the test of whether mild, non-destructive currents temporarily inhibit the tremor or rigidity (Riklan and Diller, 1961). The basal ganglia and the thalamus are the regions involved. Although subcortical mechanisms are not our explicit concern it is essential that they be mentioned to dispel the impression that only the cortex regulates these functions.

The simple picture of language representation is one which supposes that it is an exclusive left hemisphere function. The wealth of evidence discussed in a previous section shows that the left plays a major part in all speech and language functions but it suggests also that the right makes a contribution. There is evidence of subcortical involvement. The evidence of equipotentiality is something also which needs to be considered, suggesting as it does the implication of both hemispheres during critical phases of language acquisition. The picture in respect of many non-language functions is one of an interplay between one hemisphere and the other, and the two hemispheres appear to be involved in a dialogue. Something of this interaction may still occur in respect of language although the contribution from each hemisphere may by no means be equal.

There is evidence that language is not lost but that commonly speech is distorted after left cerebral lesion. The adult aphasic patient does not generally lose the language habits of a lifetime in the sense that one loses a memory and although some patients utter only a few words many retain considerable linguistic capacity. Distortions are imposed upon the customary speech habits. Many aphasics show a spontaneous recovery within a period of three to five months (Lenneberg, 1967) and there are good reasons for suspecting some reorganization of brain function. If one hemisphere can take over from the other in childhood the question remains as to whether some potential persists in the adult for the reinstatement and transfer of speech mechanisms. Also we may suspect that linguistic capacities as distinct from the mechanism of speech output are often preserved and that their presence as part of the system for general behavioural control represents a persistent and stable feature of both right and left hemisphere function. The distinction between the speech mechanisms and the capacity for linguistic ordering envisaged as two separate but interrelated systems leads us some way towards a hypothesis about language function based on the view that circumscribed lesions of the left hemisphere produce distortion but seldom total loss of speech, and that the right hemisphere also makes a contribution.

The speech process can be represented symbolically as a chain of interconnected events. The linguistic processes form the antecedent links in the chain whereas the speech output processes comprise the final links. Output systems should not be envisaged as a simple connection between the brain and the afferent neurones, however. Evidence exists of highly complex neuronal arrangements each controlling sub-patterns of the musculature. In addition there are intricate feedback networks which in their turn direct impulses into the pattern of neuromuscular flux. Output functions also comprise the selection of appropriate neuromuscular patterns in response to commands as well as in respect of the serial ordering of behaviour elements. The analogy of highly complex computing equipment is apt here The output system is the one which acts under the instruction of the linguistic codes to translate commands into the neuromuscular patterns of articulated speech.

It is clear that the output mechanisms may suffer derangement in the finer detail of control. Shankweiler *et al.* (1968) report, for example, that articulatory defects rather than reduced vocabulary or errors of syntax constitute the chief residual impairment in many patients with cortical lesion as the result of stroke in the left cerebral hemisphere. The patients are unable to form the words with sufficient accuracy and speed and it is clear from these studies that the capacity to articulate is one which when disturbed has far-reaching consequences for the production of the whole speech sequence and in more severe cases or those having not yet recovered, the articulatory difficulty itself must be expected to account for a large proportion of the language deficit.

It may be that output functions have an even greater significance. Chomsky (1964) states that there are several undemonstrated assumptions underlying the view that the speaker's behaviour should be modelled by one sort of system and the hearer's by another. McNeilage (1970) has argued, following on from Lashley's treatment of the problem of serial ordering of behaviour (Lashley, 1951), that it is possible to provide an account of the serial ordering process directly responsible for the sequencing of the movements of speech (and therefore the sounds of language).

Liberman (1957) had earlier expressed the view that articulatory movements and their sensory representations are important not only in speech but also in speech perception. Articulatory movements form building blocks which are assembled in sequence. The complex transformations of speech are cast in these same units. Sounds, it is held, are perceived by reference to the articulatory movements which produce them (Liberman *et al.*, 1963). Stimuli from the same phoneme class evoke the same mediating response and acquire similarity, whereas stimuli from different phoneme classes are distinguished by their different proprioceptive returns (Studdert-Kennedy *et al.*, 1970). Thus a theory is proposed which has great economy in that it suggests that the same system employed in output is the one also used in perception. It is not necessary at this stage to enter into the debate which has surrounded this theory except to say that there appear to be convincing grounds for supposing a close relationship of this kind. Output functions may not only generate speech from linguistic processes but those same functions may be employed to understand spoken or written language.

A number of consequences would be expected to follow from any interference with the speech output system. Dysphasia occurs after interference with lower order control mechanisms and clinically detectable aphasia from interference with the system acting to select words for articulation. Depending on the site of lesion, such interference could also disturb language perception because it disturbs the output mechanism (MacNeilage, 1970). It is to be expected that the speech output systems are located usually in the left hemisphere. There are, however, a diversity of symptoms in aphasia and lesions in endless variety implicating different areas and in different patterns will add greatly to the complexity of the symptomatology observed.

The speech systems can be viewed as the means of translating the linguistic capacities into articulated movements. The linguistic capacities, unlike the speech output systems, can be hypothesized as a feature of each hemisphere. It commonly happens that known specializations of the right come to be expressed through speech. What happens, for example, if a person should be required to use speech to describe a map or a picture? The right hemisphere is implicated with the spatial analysis, and the left with the control of speech. We might expect the right to code its analysis in terms of its own linguistic code and to direct this to the speech output system for translation into articulated sounds. Similarly we might expect the person who sings to employ the linguistic capacities of one hemisphere to express them through the speech output system of the other. There could also be high level right hemisphere contributions to the organization and planning of the speech process. The left not only contains the speech output system but also the major linguistic capacities and it should not be suggested that the left is responsible for the former and the right the latter; this is a picture which does not accord with the facts.

It seems possible that the antecedent parts of the language chain are represented in both hemispheres and that the functions of each are closely integrated. At present we know little about these more advanced functions and the problems await systematic analysis. Much of the clinical evidence can be explained, however, by the view that the speech output system and the major linguistic capacities reside in the left hemisphere in the right-handed person, but that some duplication of linguistic function occurs in the right hemisphere and there may be an interaction between the two. First, there is the evidence of equipotentiality in infancy, secondly the evidence that some language disturbances occur with right hemisphere lesions. Finally there is the

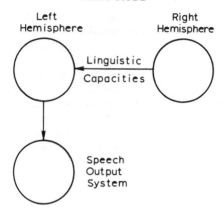

Fig. 20. Hypothetical model of right and left hemisphere contributions to the speech process.

overwhelming evidence of left hemisphere involvement. In the case of left hemisphere lesions not only may the linguistic functions suffer but damage to the speech output mechanism will interfere not only with the expression of the linguistic functions of that hemisphere, but also with any of those of the right.

CONCLUSIONS

In the view expressed by Lashley (1951) it is possible to regard the sequencing and coordination of behaviour segments as a form of grammar, having both syntactic and linguistic features. This is true irrespective of the mode of expression. Besides being expressed through the vocal apparatus or through the mechanisms of speech, grammar can be expressed through bodily movements or the movements of the limbs. In other words we have to differentiate between the speech output system and the linguistic capacities which lie beyond this system, as we may distinguish between the computer which processes the data and selects the appropriate elements and the computer programmer who channels this activity along prearranged lines.

In discussing cortical contributions to language, it is useful to distinguish between the speech processes and antecedent linguistic capacities. Sperry (1968) has shown that the right hemisphere retains little capacity for speech after section of the corpus callosum, but still displays some linguistic capacity when this is tested by means other than those employing speech. Evidence of language disturbances associated with right hemisphere lesion suggest that interference with linguistic capacity may be attributed to this source. The possibility of large-scale compensation by one hemisphere following damage to the other is something which must be considered. Lesions which might otherwise have disproportionately serious consequences may be attenuated in their effect. For example, the language deficits associated with right hemisphere lesion may represent those functions for which the left cannot adequately substitute, or those which as a matter of course employ and are dependent upon bilateral contributions. These are functions which presumably operate for the most part at the very limits of capacity that the individual is called on to perform.

It would seem from the evidence quoted here that both hemispheres are involved in linguistic capacities. Hemisphere damage to the right and the left leads to a deterioration. In the case of the left there are substantial additional deficits. These it is believed are related to interference with the speech output mechanisms, the system which translates the linguistic commands into the articulations of the speech musculature. This is a complex system responsible not only for the regulation of speech sounds, but also for the representation of linguistic codes in the choice of words and the ordering of sentences. Damage to this output system results in readily observed speech pathology. Speech remains but is disordered, although often the patient shows little additional disability. This suggests that left hemisphere damage can disrupt the speech output system, viewed as the intermediary employed to translate linguistic codes into articulated words.

Finally there is the possibility that speech may be only one means of expression of the linguistic code and that, of itself, is not necessarily the medium for higher mental processes. Other body systems having both grammar and syntax may provide alternative vehicles of communication.

9

Hemisphere Relationships

INTRODUCTION

In this chapter we not only compare the capacities of the two hemispheres, but also examine the relationship which exists between them. It is no longer sufficient to allocate functions to each. We must attempt to understand something of the working relationship between one hemisphere and the other.

Immediate difficulties are encountered in specifying the nature of the chain of command. Does control rest in the hemisphere initiating the behavioural act, or in the hemisphere supplying the information which formed the original stimulus for the initiation of the act? To a large extent we appear to be the victims of the oversimplified approach which is content to label a function and then ascribe it to either the right or the left hemisphere. But this leaves the essential problems unsolved. Naming a function is not the same thing as explaining the operation of that function, and ascribing it to one hemisphere or the other represents a type of all-or-nothing thinking which does a disservice to the statistical structure of many results.

The concept of hemisphere interrelationships has changed considerably over time. Through much of recorded history the hemispheres were regarded as identical twins. Not only did each physically resemble the other, but each was believed to match the functions of the other. With the advent of studies of speech localization the concept of cerebral dominance developed. One hemisphere came to be regarded as superordinate and the other as mute and automatic.

During recent years as more and more functions have been shown to relate predominantly to the right hemisphere, the idea of unilateral cerebral dominance has given place to the idea that one hemisphere is dominant for some functions and that the other hemisphere is dominant for others. The concept of dominance has been used liberally to mean a variety of things and the exact significance if any which it retains as a phenomenon of brain organization is a question for debate.

Most modern authors are sensitive to the need to reflect concepts of brain function accurately in the terminology they employ. The term functional pre-eminence or hemisphere differentiation can be employed to describe an association of function which is greater for one hemisphere than the other without necessarily excluding participation of the other. For instance, the left hemisphere is sometimes described as the language hemisphere. The evidence for the association is clear and yet lesions of the right hemisphere also contribute to language disturbance. This variance then may represent different parts of the language process. Even for the most clearly lateralized abilities it may be necessary to reassess the functional contribution of each hemisphere.

EARLY VIEWS OF BRAIN FUNCTION

Before the advent of the cerebral dominance view it was customary to regard the human brain as a structure in which not only was there morphological equivalence between the hemispheres but also equivalence of function. Hippocrates (c. 400 B.C.) as quoted by Chadwick and Mann (1950) commented on the duality of the human brain, pointing out that it too is double as in the case of all other animals. Gall and Spurzheim also in their catalogue of functions adopted a strictly symmetrical scheme for the localization of function. Each propensity of the mind was bilaterally represented and this indicated something of current thought at that time about hemisphere functions.

Wigan (1844) argued that the 'possession of a mind' requires only one hemisphere and that having two hemispheres makes possible the possession of two minds. Wigan regarded himself as being able to prove that each cerebrum is distinct and perfect, 'whole as an organ of thought', and that 'a separate and distinct process of thinking or ratiocination may be carried on in each cerebrum simultaneously'. Wigan described one autopsy which he performed himself in which one hemisphere was entirely gone, but it was evident that the patient, a man about 50 years of age, had conversed rationally and even written verses within a few days of his death. He describes another patient in which 'one brain was entirely destroyed—gone, annihilated, and in its place a yawning chasm'. All of his mental facilities were apparently quite perfect. Wigan finally concluded that 'one brain be a perfect instrument of thought—if it be capable of all the emotion, sentiments and faculties which we call in the aggregate mind—then it necessarily follows that man must have two minds with two brains, and however intimate and perfect their unison in their natural state, they must occasionally be discrepant when influenced by disease, either direct, sympathetic or reflex'.

Brown-Sequard (1877) supported this view of the double brain and concluded that in fact there are two brains, perfectly distinct one from the other. Ferrier (1886) also commented on the duality of the human brain. He states that 'the brain as an organ of motion and sensation or presentative consciousness is a single organ composed of two halves; the brain as an organ of ideation or representative consciousness is a dual organ, each hemisphere complete in itself. Horseley also expressed the view that we are not single animals; we are really two individuals joined together in the middle line. There is thus an early history of the view of the brain as a double system stretching back to the earliest recorded observations. Whilst we may respect the duality of structure it is apparent that although there may be considerable duplication, each half of the human brain is not an exact mirror image of the other in function. There are differences which disguise the duality although the basic double pattern may still be observed. Our task is to discuss something of these differences in an atempt to assess the significance they have for our interpretation of hemisphere relationships.

CEREBRAL DOMINANCE

The development of asymmetry of function is regarded by some authors as one of the features which differentiate the human brain from that of lower animals. Tschirgi (1958) argues that evolution consists of increasing bodily asymmetry. Man is presumed to be reaching the final category of asymmetry although at the same time it is acknowledged that he has just begun to develop a functional difference between the two hemispheres. Scheibel and Scheibel (1962) suggest that the emergence of man's highest functions are a concomitant of the nonparity of the hemispheres and they say: 'Does the emerging functional dominance of one hemisphere herald the obsolescence of the two-brained system?' This chapter sets out to suggest that the two-brained system is far from obsolete. Furthermore in reassessing the nature of cerebral dominance it sets out to show that the picture of unilateral control suggested by the theory is an exaggerated one. Young (1962) in discussing hemisphere arrangements suggests a similar view when he states that although the non-dominant hemisphere may be a vestige, personally he would prefer to keep his than lose it, and that maybe it is the two together that make the most truly useful representation of the world, partly map-like, partly abstract'.

Before discussing the arguments for and against cerebral dominance as a concept we must examine its origins more closely. Dax has been cited as originating the view that the two cerebral hemispheres are not equipotential as far as language functions are concerned and whilst Broca (1865) in his first publications admitted that both hemispheres might be involved with the language function, later he provided evidence for the pre-eminence of the left hemisphere in respect of this function. He came to the conclusion that his cases of aphemia resulted from lesion of the left half of the brain. The exceptions to this rule were soon reported, and were interpreted largely on the basis of left-handedness. Broca himself supposed that a certain number of left-handed people used the right hemisphere when speaking. 'One can conceive that there may be a certain number of individuals in whom the natural pre-eminence of the convolutions of the right hemisphere reverses the order of the phenomenon which I have just described.' Jackson (1874) took up the idea that the left hemisphere was principally concerned with speech, but with reservations. He ascribed the defects in self-expression to the left brain lesion, whilst at the same time regarding the utterances of an aphasic patient as due to the operation of the opposite intact hemisphere. Jackson regarded the right hemisphere as responsible for the 'automatic' use of words, and the left hemisphere as the leading hemisphere concerned with the creative aspects of language. However, interest was almost exclusively devoted to the association of speech with the functions of the left hemisphere. Then at a later time the facts of speech lateralization and the fact that the majority of the population are right-handed became linked together in the formulation of the concept that one hemisphere is dominant over the other. Control exercised over behaviour through thought was supposed to be inseparable from language, and the suggestion grew that one hemisphere is pre-eminent whilst the other is largely automatic and uncomprehending in its functions.

Following from this work it was generally taken to mean that speech is exclusively controlled by the left hemisphere with certain notable exceptions.

When Henschen (1926) specifically considered the right hemisphere in his review he allowed it only a compensatory role. 'Even then in every case the right hemisphere shows a manifest inferiority as compared with the left and plays an automatic role only.' In Henschen's view the right hemisphere was probably a 'regressing organ' although 'it is possible that the right hemisphere is a reserve organ'. Henschen (1926) was not entirely convinced, however, that some potential did not remain in the right hemisphere and he speculated on its role as a 'reserve organ', and as he puts it 'the hope of . . . the intelligence of future generations'.

A variety of more modern authors support a similar view. Brain (1941) supposed that it was the posterior half of the left cerebral hemisphere which formed the site of those neuronic linkages which underlie the elaboration of meanings in response to auditory and verbal stimuli and Russell and Espir (1961) supposed that the processing of past and present information arriving in the dominant hemisphere provided a scaffolding on which thought activity depends.

The observations of Liepmann (1900), Gerstmann (1927) and others on apraxia led to an extension of the concept of cerebral dominance and to its greater acceptance. Something of the quality of the different functions attributable to the different hemispheres is apparent in Schlesinger's (1962) distinction between the dominant and the subsidiary sphere of mention where he supposes a division of labour within the highest level of the neuraxis into two spheres of activity.

Dominant mentation comprises the totality of mental processes which are represented in the overt (conscious) system of notation. These are concerned with the recording of stimuli, with the elaboration of perceptions to configurations and concepts and the selection (determination of responses). The subsidiary sphere of mentation on the other hand does not record stimuli directly and it uses for the purpose of the determination of response data represented in the mnemonic rather than the overt system of notation.

The cerebral dominance viewpoint has its contemporary supporters. Indeed a rearguard action has been fought around the supposition that as the right hemisphere plays no special role, brain lesions tend to be larger in this area because the surgeon is less sparing of tissue with the consequence of greater deficits in performance. This may be the case although we may be reluctant to accept that full value is not placed on any form of brain tissue as this argument implies. Even if this is so however it is still possible to argue that for the removal of brain tissue to have an effect it must conduct important functions, and the fact that removal produces the effect at all shows that the tissue plays some part in the regulation of behaviour.

Various descriptions of the role of the cerebral hemispheres have been provided in the light of the cerebral dominance concept. Anderson (1951) summarized the results of his investigations. When the minor is injured one can say that it forgets what it ought to do, when the dominant is injured one can say that it no longer knows how to do it. Hécaen et al. suggest that the dominant hemisphere is responsible for the execution of activities and that the minor hemisphere creates the conditions necessary for their execution. They quote Pierre and Hoff (1950) who suggest that the role of the left hemisphere would be to construct new functional schemata in relation to the higher human activities and performance, while the role of the right hemisphere would consist in the preparation of the means for accomplishing these performances by supplying the correct temporal ideas, and by assessing the overall situation of the body and relations in space.

SOME OBJECTIONS TO THE CONCEPT OF
CEREBRAL DOMINANCE

Although the concept of cerebral dominance may appear to explain the facts of brain function, there are objections to it and the concept now has to be viewed more critically. An attempt has been made to appraise the problem previously (Dimond, 1970b, 1971b). Evidence for the view that one hemisphere predominates in function rests both on the facts of handedness and on the facts of the lateralization of speech. The large majority of the population are right-handed, the minority are left-handed. The possibility of substantial representation amongst the population of mixed handers is one which needs to be considered seriously (Annett, 1964).

Not only may the right-handed person prefer to use his right hand but he may also prefer to use his right foot and to a lesser extent his right eye. In calling into question the value of some aspects of the cerebral dominance standpoint it is not the intention to dispute these facts of laterality. The right hand or limb is dominant in that it is preferred over the left when the individual is required to choose, but in other respects the picture is by no means so clear. The right hand is not always the superior when comparison is made of individual performance (Provins, 1967). It can be argued that disproportional significance has attributed to the concept of hand dominance because the performance of the two hands may resemble one another to an extent which far outweighs the difference between them.

Hand dominance is something which is not seriously questioned here, however, although certain reservations may have to be made. The question of the functional superiority of one hemisphere over the other is our present concern. The cerebral dominance viewpoint supposes that because the right hand is employed in preference to the left, the hemisphere controlling the functions of the right hand must therefore be dominant and the hemisphere controlling the functions of the left the subordinate. It is not possible to deny the preference for the right hand over the left and equally it cannot be denied that each hand maintains a special anatomical link to the contralateral hemisphere. Stimulation of the precentral gyrus evokes limb movement on the contralateral side.

The question arises however as to the relationship between the hand and the controlling hemisphere. It is true to say that hand dominance is not the same thing as hemisphere dominance. The hand is in a sense the messenger of the hemisphere. Control of the hand is one, but only one of the functions carried out by the hemisphere. There is some case to be made out for divorcing hemisphere function from hand function. Although we might expect a relationship between the hemisphere and the hand it does not follow that it is of a one-to-one topological kind.

We now have to question in more detail the assumptions that the superiority of one hemisphere over the other is revealed by that of the functions of the limbs.

It is the case that there are numerous interconnecting systems between one hemisphere and the other. The subcortical mechanisms allow one to contact the other, and the neocortical commissures permit a continuous interplay in the day-to-day regulation of the functions of the brain. It is difficult to think of the cerebral hemispheres as functioning in isolation. We cannot regard the accomplishments of the right hand as determined exclusively by the decisions of the left hemisphere, neither can we regard those of the left as determined exclusively by the right. If we take a very simple example, that of threading a needle, the neural processes on this simple task are not confined separately and exclusively to each hemisphere. Both must be in a state of flux directing and redirecting messages across the brain to achieve the necessary coordination. We have to consider that one hemisphere can work through another as well as the evident fact that each may integrate functions with the other. We are thus led to question if control can be regarded as confined exclusively to the one hemisphere to which the hand is linked. The view expressed here is not the one which supposes that the whole brain is implicated in any function in Gestalt fashion, but it is accepted that control may reside at more distant parts of the brain than at the output system to the hand.

Control of the functions of the hands is more complicated than the cerebral dominance viewpoint would lead us to suppose but what is the significance of the difference between one hand and the other? It has been suggested previously (Chapter 7) that the motor output system to the right is more sophisticated than that to the left (Dimond, 1970b). The motor output system is highly complex, a network of systems and sub-systems with intricate feedback and control mechanisms (Hinde, 1966). If we attribute behavioural phenomena to lower order neural mechanisms before seeking explanation at other levels we should investigate motor output systems first. The elevated performance of the limb would reflect the action of a motor system of greater proficiency—it would also come to be preferred over the other.

Neuromuscular laterality can be regarded as a specialization of the brain relating to the left hemisphere but at the same time it is not necessary to conclude from evidence of handedness that one hemisphere controls the functions of the other. The motor system mediates between the brain and the external world. At the same time it need not be viewed as the source of the decisions which it operates.

The second relationship to be considered is that of speech to cerebral dominance. The history of this has been discussed previously. There is an unequivocal association of speech with the left hemisphere. At the same time there is increasing evidence which suggests that the right hemisphere is to some extent involved. The hypothesis was advanced in a previous chapter that both hemispheres play some part in the antecedent events of the language chain, but that at the same time the output system which acts to select words and to place them in their correct sequence resides in the left hemisphere only. Both hemispheres apparently play some part in the genesis of language but the left plays its part through linguistic means and the lateralization of the mechanisms of output control.

In the past the idea has been prevalent that language has unique properties. Language is the vehicle for the control of behaviour, language is the mechanism of thought, and internal speech forms the inner substance of the mental life. All of these activities were attributed to the left hemisphere because of its association with speech. If the right hemisphere is also important however in relation to linguistic formulation even if not to speech output, the ascription of higher mental processes exclusively to the left becomes more difficult.

In the early days it appeared reasonable to suppose that the left hemisphere was dominant on the basis of evidence available at that time. The original formulations are however no longer as tenable because of the evidence which shows that left hemisphere superiority in respect of some functions can be matched by right hemisphere superiority for others. The evidence for right hemisphere superiority will be reviewed under the heading of hemisphere differentiation. At this stage it is sufficient to point to the fact that the right hemisphere displays superiority in respect of some visual and auditory functions, visuo-spatial and constructive abilities, and musical capacities. The demonstration that the left does not exercise exclusive superiority over all functions has led modern writers to support a modified concept of cerebral dominance which tends to be related to the function under consideration. According to this view, dominance can change from one hemisphere to another and is not exclusive to one.

It has been the custom to regard the hemispheres as isolated units but the possibility of one hemisphere working through another has to be considered. The work cited earlier on investigation of function after section of the corpus callosum suggests bilateral representation in respect of numerous functions but it also suggests that the hemispheres are in close contact normally by virtue of crosstalk over the corpus callosum and other midline transport systems. Evidence for intercommunication has focused attention on the power of the cerebral hemispheres to interact. Dimond (1970b) has suggested that one hemisphere, either the right or the left, can form the vehicle through which the other can express specialized capacities. The language output centre of the left hemisphere could for example be employed working through the corpus callosum and the right hemisphere to enable the person to write with the left hand. Similarly the visuo-spatial capacities of the right hemisphere again passing through the corpus callosum and the left hemisphere could be expressed when the right hand is used in drawing or in other types of visuo spatial construction. In fact Gazzaniga et al. (1965) report that a patient who had formerly been able to draw well using the right hand lost most of this capacity after section of the callosum, but could draw well with the left. This suggests that the concept of cerebral dominance as unilateral control of one hemisphere by another needs some reappraisal. In its place it could be suggested that areas of special capacity are cross-linked to motor output areas as the need arises, and that such links are utilized at the command of either hemisphere.

HEMISPHERE DIFFERENTIATION

COMPARISON OF HEMISPHERE FUNCTION

The concept of exclusive unilateral cerebral dominance has given place to one which is truly bilateral but differs according to different functions. Dominance can be attributed to one hemisphere in respect of one function, but may at the same time be attributed to another for another function. Thus Nielson (1946) speaks of the major hemisphere and the minor hemisphere for given functions, wishing to indicate by this a simple quantitative difference in the potential of symmetrical zones. In recent years we have seen many studies in which functions are compared. The results in some cases show that each hemisphere makes an equal contribution; some show the left and others the right to be superior.

Cases are reported which show no significant differences between the hemispheres but because of a perspective which only seeks to find differences these results are often overlooked. There is an impairment of function, but this is equal and opposite between the hemispheres. Such results are of interest however if a view is adopted that the human brain is largely a bilateral system although acknowledging that hemisphere differences may be superimposed over this. Abilities in which the interference of a lesion has been found to be equal and opposite are those of tactile size judgment (Weinstein, 1955a), weight judgment (Weinstein, 1955b), the perception of hidden figures (Teuber and Weinstein, 1954), performances on complex tactual tasks, spatial orientation (Semmes *et al.*, 1955) and tactile discrimination (Ghent *et al.*, 1955) and many others. Indeed we might expect a deterioration on both sides to be frequent. When personality disturbances are considered it has been reported also by Hécaen (1962) that no differences are to be found in cases with right and left hemisphere lesion, although at the same time the evidence is somewhat equivocal on this point (Semmes *et al.*, 1960).

LEFT HEMISPHERE

Evidence in respect of left hemisphere differentiation for language has been discussed in a previous chapter and there is little need to elaborate on it here. There are a number of additional associated deficits, memory for example. Meyer and Yates (1955) showed that there is a disturbance in the recall of verbal material which accompanies lesion of the left temporal lobe in tasks of associative learning. Milner (1962) also reports a similar deficit for a test of story recall and quotes evidence from subtests of the Wechsler Memory Scale to support the view that there is a verbal memory difficulty in patients with epileptogenic lesions of the left temporal lobe (Milner, 1956).

Intelligence tests have been used to measure language deficit; by and large these show a deficit in verbal intelligence which accompanies left hemisphere lesion. Anderson (1951) for example administered the Wechsler Bellvue Intelligence scale to individuals with right or left hemisphere lesions and reported a significantly greater loss of verbal function with left hemisphere lesions and a significantly greater loss for nonverbal function with right hemisphere lesions. There have been a number of confirmatory reports (Costa and Vaughan, 1962; Stark, 1961).

Parsons *et al.* (1969) also using the vocabulary test and the block design test of the WAIS showed that right hemisphere damage results in impaired visuo-constructive performance and left hemisphere damage affects language abilities. The tendency to classify abilities into either one of two types, verbal or spatial—the classification of the Wechsler Bellvue Intelligence scale—can be potentially misleading in that labelling a factor is not the same thing as explaining it. Also abilities may be regarded as separate when there can be elements in common.

RIGHT HEMISPHERE

Little was known until recently about the functions of the right hemisphere. The problems of hemisphere control appear in a different light when consideration is given to the fact that the right hemisphere is also differentiated and that it also has its own special province.

Teuber (1962) for example states that it becomes increasingly probable that right hemispheric lesions in man may alter perception in a different way from the case where there are lesions on the left side. Teuber studied the effects of penetrating cerebral lesions in previously healthy adults to understand something of how fairly stable lesions in the nervous system might bring an understanding of cerebral pathology. Some of the expected differences between the hemispheres were immediately apparent. Lesions of the left hemisphere, particularly those of the left parietotemporal region, produced significant and lasting losses on a (predominantly verbal) test of general intelligence. Such changes are well documented and need not concern us here.

What does concern us are the effects of right hemisphere lesions perhaps previously categorized as complex perceptual changes or the hampering of visuo-constructive achievements (McFie, Piercy and Zangwill, 1950). This type of deficit after right hemispheric lesion has been revealed using pictorial material (Milner, 1954; Cohen, 1959; Landsell, 1961).

The contribution of the right hemisphere to spatial perception was suggested earlier by Jackson (1876). He states: 'I think that the posterior lobes are the seat of the most intellectual processes. This is in effect saying that they are the seat of visual ideation, for most of our mental operations are carried on in visual ideals. I think too that the right posterior lobe is the leading side, the left the more automatic.'

Following Jackson's observations case histories were published suggesting that the right hemisphere was critically involved in spatial perception. These were reviewed by Lange (1936) and others who all emphasized the importance of the right parieto-occipital region. Lange (1936) commented that right hemisphere disorders were of 'surprisingly' great importance for spatial skills, both in their visual and constructional aspects as if the right hemisphere provides the ground or foundation of the world image.

Evidence of a spatial deficit following right hemisphere lesions has now accumulated from a substantial number of investigations (Hebb, 1939; Paterson and Zangwill, 1944; Piercy and Smyth, 1962; Warrington and James, 1967), and deficits in constructional capacities have been reported after right hemispherectomy (Griffith and Davidson, 1966). The contribution of the right hemisphere in cases of disturbance of body image has been reported. Brain (1941) described a symptom of neglect of one side of the visual field and space connected with that field following right hemisphere lesion. McFie, Piercy and Zangwill (1950) also established that lesions of the non-dominant hemisphere could give rise to disturbances of spatial perception and of constructive activities; this was later confirmed by Hécaen (1959). Hécaen (1962) also describes cases of apraxia which stem from a right hemisphere symptomology. Apraxia for dressing for example can follow as a consequence of right sided retro-Rolandic lesions. The apraxic syndrome due to non-dominant hemisphere lesions is characterized by two essential elements, in the first place a visuo-constructive disorder and in the second place apraxia for dressing (Arrigoni and De Renzi, 1964).

A disorder of spatial thought is often associated with bilateral or diffuse brain disease but it can also occur when the injury is restricted to one hemisphere alone (Critchley, 1953). Nielsen (1946) showed a marked association of disorders of spatial thought associated with the right occipital lobe, and was led to conclude that the right occipital lobe is dominant far more often than would be anticipated on the basis of left-handedness. Benton (1967) also showed that some of the effects which have been found in patients with unilateral post-Rolandic lesions are demonstrable in patients with unilateral frontal lesions. The generalization holds for verbal tests as well as for tests of constructional apraxia which again revealed an association with right hemisphere functions.

Some relationship of the right hemisphere to the triggering of what has been described as 'visual fits' is in evidence. Penfield (1958) reports that 10 out of 11 cases showing epileptic attacks either beginning with visual manifestations or entirely confined to the visual sphere have right temporal lesions. Hécaen and Badaracco (1956) also report that of 16 similar patients, 14 seemed to have a lesion in the right rather than the left hemisphere. Teuber, Battersby and Bender (1960) report in their group of similar missile wound patients that 13 of the 15 had wounds implicating the right hemisphere. Déjà-vu phenomena are also more frequently experienced by patients with right hemisphere lesions (Cole and Zangwill, 1963). Results of this kind are not conclusive because of the nature of the disorder but they suggest that the right hemisphere may have some primacy in the organization of visual function, and it is tempting to regard them as supporting earlier contentions of the right hemisphere as the primary visual organizing region.

There is some evidence that the right hemisphere might play a disproportionate part in binaural localization. With right parieto temporal lesions there can be a greater impairment of binaural localization (Teuber and Diamond, 1956). There are also evidences of a greater right hemisphere involvement in respect of the control over tactual processes. In one investigation described by Teuber and Weinstein (1954) a form board was used which required the patients to fit various blocks into the appropriate holes without vision. The form board was administered first in the original position and then after rotation through 180°. Only those with right temporal lesions showed themselves to be disturbed in their performance after the board was rotated. This pointed to a striking disturbance of learning performance on this task. Weinstein (1962) carried out a further investigation of tactile size discrimination. The subjects were required to identify three-dimensional wooden shapes by palpating them with the fingers. Patients with lesions of the central or Rolandic region of the brain and patients with right hemisphere lesions were significantly inferior in performance to controls. Weinstein showed that this deficit could not be due to a lack of sensitivity, although sensory defect contributed to it. Eleven of the 19 men with right hemisphere lesion showed the defect whereas only four of the 23 left hemisphere lesion men showed the defect. Certain nonverbal achievements may depend more markedly upon the integrity of the right than of the left hemisphere.

Milner (1968) reports that patients with right temporal lobe injury show a variety of deficits on visual non-verbal tasks. They are for example slow and inaccurate in detecting incongruities in sketchy, cartoon-like drawings. They also show a deficit in the recognition of overlapping nonsense figures and groups of dots tachistoscopically presented. There was ample evidence of visual memory defect after right temporal lobectomy but not after left temporal lobectomy (Milner, 1960; Landsell, 1961). This was shown on a face recognition procedure, and in respect of learning to recognize nonsense figures over repeated presentations, as well as in the delayed recall of geometric figures.

Luria (1963) considered the right hemisphere to be dominant in respect of a number of intellectual abilities. Musical ability was one of these, and he describes a composer whose best work was done after he became aphasic with a massive stroke in the left hemisphere. Head (1926) also described several somewhat similar patients who retained musical capacity apparently in the right hemisphere. Evidence for the association of right hemisphere function with musical ability has been extensively reviewed by Bogen (1969b).

In respect of auditory functions, Milner (1962) reports that there are some differences in time on the Seashore Time and Rhythm test following right temporal lobectomy similarly with errors in the perception of loudness, and the error scores for Timbre and Tonal memory increase markedly in patients with right temporal lesions. The results show that a right temporal lobectomy has effects on musical and non-verbal auditory tests, difficult comparisons of tonal patterns or judgments of tone quality being the most affected.

It is clear that with the recognition that these functions are predominantly associated with the right hemisphere, old ideas of cerebral dominance as exclusively unilateral are no longer acceptable.

Hécaen (1962) suggests that 'the facts so far generated suggest that there exists a specific symptomatology for each hemisphere, without so far having the right to infer from that the existence of particular functions. It is a fact that the symptomatology is different according to the hemisphere disturbed thus obliging us to consider a certain functional organization of the cortex that would be different for each hemisphere'.

Several authors suggest that one hemisphere is dominant for some functions and that the other hemisphere is dominant for others. Kreindler *et al.* (1966) suggest for example that 'Each function presents a certain autonomy and is not inevitably lateralized to a particular hemisphere. Although in the majority of right handers the left hemisphere is dominant for motricity and language, for visuo-spatial orientation there is a dominance of the right hemisphere.

The theory of hemisphere differentiation assigns qualitatively distinct roles in performance to each hemisphere. It supposes in essence that each has unique functions to perform and that each in its own way is specialized for control. This is an extension of the principle of dominance assumed by one hemisphere at one time and by the other at another. In this sense the ideas are quite far removed from the traditional unilateral construct. The concepts of hemisphere differentiation approach more closely the picture of brain function revealed by contemporary research. There is a tendency still to regard the hemisphere evidencing the superiority as the one which bears the exclusive responsibility for this function. This is once again an all or none approach which in most instances does not accord with the statistical structure of the data. Zangwill (1960) allows for the possibility of some although unequal representation to both hemispheres where this is necessitated in the phrase 'functional pre-eminence'.

Even in respect of hemisphere differentiation it is possible that greater significance attaches to the concept of dominance than it may warrant. Slight but significant differences can appear in the results of investigations which lead the investigator to conclude that one hemisphere is dominant over the other. However, the similarities may outweigh any difference in performance and the latter contributes only to a limited extent to the total variance of the situation. The more serious objection is that although one hemisphere may be shown to be dominant, we may still be unable to assess the significance of what this means as regards the control of behaviour.

Finally we may have to accept the view that many kinds of complex relationships are possible, and that the propensity of each hemisphere to develop patterns of lawful control over behaviour suggests that there is also a suprastructure of control lying over and above the lateralized functions. The controlling suprastructure cross- switches or links the localized areas to the bodily mechanisms.

The view supported here has been described as a middle of the road interpretation (Benton, 1964), it asserts that while both hemispheres play a qualitative role, the contribution of one may be more important than the contribution of the other in respect of certain performances. At the same time weight must be given to the interplay between one hemisphere and the other and the integration of functions each within the performances of the other. This is envisaged largely as a cross-switching system by which the functions of each side of the body are able to gain access to the areas of specialization within each hemisphere.

CONCLUSIONS

In this chapter we have traced the progress of ideas about hemisphere relationships through early concepts that each hemisphere is the exact mirror image of the other in respect to function, that complete unilateral control exists to more modern ideas that one may be superior for some functions and the other superior for other functions.

At the same time it is pointed out that this may not be an all or none affair. Considerable redundancy may operate in hemispheric control, and the effects of lesions may reflect a situation in which supplementary compensation is no longer possible. The concept of dominance has a limited use for it does not explain how it is that behavioural control is established. It is a descriptive term which ties a particular function to a particular hemisphere, without explaining how that function is generated. It may be misleading because it can suggest unilateral function when a view of bilateral though unequal contributions may be more relevant.

It is therefore advisable to examine the situation afresh and to recognize the need for flexibility in the system. It is suggested that cross-switching systems may operate so that different capacities can be expressed in different ways. It is important to remember that each cerebral hemisphere is not an isolated unit, and to understand behaviour it may be of only limited importance to know that one hemisphere is superior in any one function. What is much more important is to understand something of the complex cross-talk between the two hemispheres and to study the continual interplay which determines the control of behaviour.

10

Conclusions

INTRODUCTION

This book has gathered together from a wide variety of fields information relating to the two-brain organization. Evidence about the tandem arrangement of the cerebral hemispheres came from studies of brain lesion in man and animal, and from studies of hemispherectomy and section of the corpus callosum. It also examined the behaviour of the normal person.

From these sources it is possible to draw three overall conclusions. The first is that the two-brain interpretation is valid both for the nervous system of man and for that of lower animals. Secondly, that the bilateral arrangement allows the total productive capacity of the brain to be increased. Thirdly, that the hemispheres do not work in an all or none fashion, but take part in a highly integrated fusion of functions which is mediated largely by the transporting action of the corpus callosum.

THE TWO-BRAIN SYSTEM IN ACTION

From a diffuse and composite network, we witness the progressive development of nervous mechanisms towards a double system. In its origins the nervous system consists of not many, but two lateral nerve cords each accompanied by cerebral ganglia. This double feature is preserved in the brain of higher vertebrates including man. The pattern was set early in evolutionary history and has persisted throughout representative species including man. The infra-human species possesses a double brain in which each hemisphere is the mirror image of the other, both in structure and function.

Studies of spreading cortical depression show that each hemisphere has the capacity to perceive, to remember, and to learn independently of the other; each is equipped to control behaviour even in the absence of its companion; and each bears the same stamp for acquisition performance. But although each duplicates the other in respect of all major functions, the performance of the single hemisphere does not completely match that of the two-brain system. There is evidence to suggest that two hemispheres can work together and perform better than one.

The findings of bilateral representation in the animal brain are confirmed by studies of hemispherectomy. removal of one hemisphere, whilst not leaving the animal unaffected, does not have as serious consequences as might at first be supposed. Each hemisphere can take over functions of the other, and after a time the organism may appear to function almost as well with one as with two hemispheres. There is very little evidence of asymmetry in brain function and no substantial evidence that one hemisphere exclusively directs the functions of the other. The arrangement appears to be a true partnership with much additional duplication of function.

Motor disturbances accompany hemispherectomy in both animals and man. If there is early brain damage, the disturbances after removal of the right hemisphere resemble those after removal of the left with the exception that they are located in the opposite half of the body. Motor representation occurs as a double system controlled in a bilateral fashion. One hemisphere appears to substitute for a variety of functions when the other is removed. These functions include that of learned reponse, in addition to those of perception and memory. There is also some potential for restitution of complex abilities.

Patients who develop cerebral pathology in one hemisphere early in life may not be greatly affected by removal of the diseased hemisphere. Until a certain age, considerable potential for the development of the complete range of human functions appears to exist in each hemisphere. There is too a remarkable preservation of intellectual ability, and the fact that consciousness persists suggests that it is not the prerogative of a single hemisphere. Studies of hemispherectomy point to the inevitable conclusion that the potential for duplication of function exists on a large scale in the human brain.

Some of the most important work supporting the concept of the two-brain system is the study of callosal section in both animals and man. The corpus callosum represents a significant and recent achievement in the evolutionary history of the brain. The callosal fibres connect corresponding points in the cerebral hemispheres, and a large measure of functional separation can be achieved by its section. Each hemisphere has the capacity to perceive, to remember, and to learn. Each can, under certain circumstances, carry out these functions independently of the other, and by sectioning the mid-brain commissures, two systems are created, which apparently function independently. Those functions which show transfer across the midline, Gazzaniga (1969) is inclined to attribute to proprioceptive movement.

He argues that head and eye movements provide information to the hand which is used to direct it towards a target.

Early investigations suggested that no important behavioural symptoms are to be observed following section of the corpus callosum in man, providing that other symptoms of brain damage are absent. Later reports (Bogen and Vogel, 1962; Bogen, Fisher and Vogel, 1965; Sperry, 1968) showed this view to be mistaken. More recent investigations have shown that without the corpus callosum, the brain appeared as 'two individuals inhabiting the same body'. The behaviour of split-brain patients suggests that the capacities for learning, remembering and perception are duplicated within each cerebral hemisphere.

Sperry (1968) says that tests indicate the presence in the right hemisphere of a special capacity 'for things like insight, mental association and ideation'. This is largely based on the ability of the right hemisphere to select items indicated by a particular instruction or associated with a particular stimulus. Although there may well be differences in capacity between the hemispheres in man, nonetheless evidence of cerebral function in split-brain patients suggests that the two-brain system is still representative even when higher mental processes, e.g. ideation, mental association or consciousness, are considered. In respect of language, the situation is rather different. The person with a split-brain is able to speak with one hemisphere but not with the other. It may be that all language processes reside in one hemisphere alone, as has been suggested in the past. Alternatively, it may be that ordering and control of speech output rests with the left hemisphere, but that linguistic potential can arise in both. It is argued here somewhat speculatively, that linguistic capacities do in fact relate to both cerebral hemispheres.

Studies of blocks to function support the view that each hemisphere possesses its own intrinsic analysing system which processes the information it receives. These studies suggest that the hemisphere proceeds a considerable distance along the chain of analysis before the possibility of sharing information with the other hemisphere arises.

Turning now to the question of laterality, it is acknowledged that there are differences in the representation of function between the two sides, though in the human brain this is not an all or none relationship. If the case of language is considered, a function which might be regarded as lateralized more than any other, we find that the left hemisphere appears to take the major share, but that the right may contribute certain complex linguistic characteristics, and possibly be involved in the planning of the speech process itself. In other words, lateralization is not exclusive. The evidence indicates a contribution from both hemispheres, representing an extension of the two-brain system of lower animals.

Thus evidence from many sources suggests that the idea that one hemisphere is non-functional or vestigial cannot be supported, and that the two-brain concept is valid both for the nervous system of lower animals and for man.

EXTENSION OF BRAIN CAPACITY

If it is asked how it is that the brain evolved as a double system, one answer must be that it did so as a response to the need to separate out and analyse independently input from different lateral regions of space. Another reason must surely be the development of control over a body which was bilaterally symmetrical. The two-brain system allowed separate control of the muscle blocks on each side, and division of the brain facilitated the link-up of stimuli from one side with muscular responses on the same side and thus directly related them to the nature of the stimulation. In evolutionary terms, there was some value in having a double system instead of one fused and undifferentiated in the mid-plane.

Independent detection of left/right stimuli also had the advantage that it permitted a separate analysis of events which can ultimately be combined and employed to perform such complex functions as distance computation or the perception of three dimensional space. It might be expected also that in combining the products of separate analysis certain advantages would be gained. The use of two brains may prove to be more efficient than the use of one, and indeed experiments suggest that two hemispheres working in harmony can extend the range of brain capacity.

Spreading cortical depression can be used to train each hemisphere separately in performing parts of a task which need to be combined to produce the final solution. When this is done, the solution may be easier to accomplish than under circumstances where normal controls are used and both hemispheres receive training on both parts of the task. Each hemisphere has the capacity to integrate with the other, so that two hemispheres are not only superior to one but also, under these conditions, to the brain of the normal animal trained with both hemispheres intact. When the task is shared between the hemispheres, performance is enhanced. This supports the view that whilst each has the capacity to learn, to remember, and to perceive, two systems may be better than one, and the limitations of achievement can be related closely to the joint action of both (Burešová and Bureš, 1969).

The evolution of a mechanisms to facilitate integration between one hemisphere and the other would appear to be a prerequisite for interchange of functions of this kind. The corpus callosum develops and expands during the course of evolution of the vertebrate nervous system, to reach imposing proportions in the brain of man. The evolution of cross-connecting fibres is undoubtedly a feature contributing to the development of the higher mental processes.

Many of the recent evolutionary achievements of the brain can be attributed to the increasing significance of the mechanisms of the corpus callosum and the cerebral commissures. In the split-brain animal it is possible to perform a totally different task. This is done without any apparent sign of conflict. Gazzaniga and Young (1968) found that the split-brain monkey can process and respond to more information involving bimanual motor sequencing, than can controls with their commissures intact. Presumably this increase in capacity stems from a greater capacity for independent function. Separation disconnects the previously cooperating machinery and divides the brain into two functioning wholes. One part of the total information necessary to solve a problem may be given to one hemisphere and another part to the other. In this case monkeys with the corpus callosum sectioned were totally unable to integrate the information from both hemispheres and performance remained at chance levels. Again, when investigations were made to test integration, the animal showed evidence that each hemisphere processed its information without knowledge of the other's functions. When both halves of the information were projected to the single hemisphere, the monkeys produced high-level solutions to the problem.

Commissurotomy patients can carry out double voluntary reaction time tasks as fast as they can carry out a single reaction (Gazzaniga and Sperry, 1966). This not only suggests that each hemisphere possesses the necessary equipment to analyse and to register signals, as well as to organize response, but also that in the normal commissure-linked hemispheres, something of this additional capacity could well remain.

If a visual discrimination task is presented first to the left hemisphere, and then the same task with another discrimination task to the right hemisphere, response times to the single and the double presentation show that there is no interference of one discrimination task with the other.

The present author's own studies of blocks to function within the nervous system support the view that in the normal person two hemispheres can accomplish more than one. The split-brain person may show doubled capacity if one stream of signals are directed to one hemisphere at the same time as another stream of signals are directed to the other hemisphere. This enhancement of performance is also characteristic of the normal brain. Although capacity may not be doubled, facilitation is observed when signal load is shared between the hemispheres. This again suggests that each hemisphere of the normal brain not only carries out an analysis of the information it receives, a function assumedly indispensable to space and distance perception, but also that the use of two hemispheres as receptive systems augments the total output achieved by the brain.

Two messages directed to separate hemispheres are registered more effectively than two messages projected to the same hemisphere. The picture of brain function observed in split-brain patients has important corollaries for the interpretation of normal human function. Such a picture points to the need to study the behaviour of normal people in the light of a two-brain system possessing duplicate mechanisms and tandem arrangements, as well as to investigate the potential for integration and subsequent interaction of function after perceptual analysis.

It is not suggested that it will be possible in the immediate future to extend brain capacity in a practical sense by the full employment of both hemispheres. Rather the view is advanced that the two-brain system allows for the development of a fuller capacity than might otherwise exist. Functions are not confined exclusively to one hemisphere, the other being a 'spare tyre' should the occasion arise, but each is an active member of the partnership and it could be envisaged that load sharing and distribution may be a prominent feature of this system. The double brain allows for isomorphic map-like representation of space. It provides a mechanism of bilateral motor control and a means by which events occuring in regions of space become linked to isomorphic lateral motor response. At the same time a double system allows for a greater capacity of perceptual analysis and this enables the organism to support a more effective relationship with the world.

FUNCTIONAL INTEGRATION

Recent investigations of the corpus callosum show that the hemispheres are not isolated units. The picture of brain function presented here is not that of the unilateral control and domination of one hemisphere by the other, neither is it that of a double system in which one hemisphere carries out duties exclusive to itself while the opposite hemisphere carries out other duties. It is of a two-brain system in which functions are to a large degree bilaterally represented, a system in which the functions of each hemisphere interlock closely with those of the other. Even a simple task like threading a needle involves a barrage of cross-talk, integrating the spatial functions with those of the limbs on both sides of the body. This continuous interplay between one hemisphere and the other is regarded as inherent in normal brain activity.

The need for integration can be seen when muscle patterns are considered. Simple movements evoke the activities of muscle synergies around the body, relaxation of some, contraction of others, and a host of additional postural adjustments. The activities of one side of the body are not separate from those of the other, they are enmeshed with them. Similarly, hemisphere functions can be viewed as interlacing systems which signal to one another through intense bursts of inter-communication.

Studies of spreading cortical depression show that the hemispheres integrate function in the ordinary course of events, to the extent of setting up replica memory models in each hemisphere. The tandem arrangement extends capacity for complex performances, and this is achieved through integration and by combining elements originally planted separately in each cerebral hemisphere. There seems little doubt that a complex interchange does take place which allows the boundaries of performance to be extended and the work of the system to be shared. Studies of split-brain function in animals suggest widespread integration of function between one hemisphere and the other by means of cross-talk over the corpus callosum. Certainly when the corpus is sectioned this kind of integration may no longer be possible, and the evidence suggests that integration is now seriously impaired.

In the patient described by Bogen and Vogel (1962) the wholeness of the corpus callosum appeared to be essential to integration of hemisphere function. It is clear, however, that even in the absence of the corpus callosum there are mechanisms by which one hemisphere finds out about the functions of the other. The possibility exists that re-routing of information takes place through the mid-brain regions. Probably the presence of extensive body feedback networks allow one hemisphere, through the product of learning, to retain close contact with the output of the other. It seems likely also that one picks up clues about the other simply by 'listening' or 'observing' what it does. The principal means of intercommunication between one and the other would still appear to be the corpus callosum and the other mid-brain commissures, and it is to these that we have to attribute ultimately the facility for intercommunication and integration of functions. One major element is that each hemisphere can signal information about its actions, both as they occur and in advance (Schaffer, 1969). We have seen that advance cortical decision potentials are a feature of intentions to act (Gilden et al., 1967). The mid-brain commissures show every likelihood of transmitting these in coded form in addition to information about acts which may already be taking place.

Functions cannot be attributed exclusively to one hemisphere or the other, and although one may take the lion's share, the important problem is not now to parcel out functions on an either/or basis, but to understand how the total output of the human brain is a function of the integration of the two hemispheres, the alter and the alterum.

References

Abrams, K. and Bever, T. G. (1969). Syntactic structure modifies attention during speech perception and recognition. *Quart. J. Exp Psychol.*, *21(3)*, 280-290.

Akelaitis, A. J. (1940). A study of gnosis, praxis and language following partial and complete section of the corpus callosum. *Trans. Amer. Neurol. Ass.*, *66*, 182-185.

Akelaitis, A. J. (1941a). Studies on corpus callosum: higher visual functions in each homonymous field following complete section of corpus callosum. *Arch. Neurol. Psychiat. (Chic.)*, 45, 788.

Akelaitis, A. J. (1941b). Studies of the corpus callosum. VIII: The effect of partial and complete section of the corpus callosum on psychopathic epileptics. *Amer. J. Psychiat.*, *98*, 409.

Akelaitis, A. J. (1942a). Studies on the corpus callosum. V: Homonymous defects for colour, object and letter recognition (homonymous hemiamblyopia) before and after section of the corpus callosum. *Arch Neurol. Psychiat. (Chic.)*, *48*, 108-118.

Akelaitis, A. J. (1942b). Studies on the corpus callosum. VI: Orientation (temporal-spatial gnosis) following section of the corpus callosum. *Arch. Neurol. Psychiat. (Chic.)*, *48*, 914-937.

Akelaitis, A. J. (1944). Study of gnosis, praxis, and language following section of corpus callosum and anterior commissure. *J. Neurosurg.*, *1*, 94.

Anderson, A. L. (1951). The effect of laterality localization on focal brain lesions on the Wechsler-Bellvue subtests. *J. Clin. Psychol.*, *7*, 149-153.

Annett, M. (1964). A model of the inheritance of handedness and cerebral dominance. *Nature (Lond.)*, *204*, 59-60.

Annett, M. (1967). The binomial distribution of right, mixed and left handedness. *Quart. J. Exp. Psychol.*, *19*, 327-333.

Ariëns Kappers, C. U., Huber, G. C. and Crosby, E. C. (1960). *The comparative anatomy of the nervous system of vertebrates including man*, vol. 3. New York: Hafner Publ. Co.

Arrigoni, G. and DeRenzi, E. (1964). Constructional apraxia and hemispheric locus of lesion. *Cortex*, *1(2)*, 170-197.

Attneave, F. (1959). Applications of information theory to psychology. New York: Henry Holt and Co.

Bailey, P. and von Bonin, G. (1951). *The isocortex of man.* Chicago: Univ. of Illinois Press.

Bakker, D. J. (1967). Left-right differences in auditory perception of verbal and non-verbal material by children. *Quart. J. Exp. Psychol.*, *19*, 334-336.

Bard, P. (1933). Studies on the cerebral cortex. I: Localized control of placing and hopping reactions in the cat and their normal management by small cortical remnants. *Arch. Neur. Psychiat.*, *30*, 40-74.

Baru, A. V. (1955). Some effects of removal of the anterior brain and the tectum optici on the conditioning of the fish (teleost). Questions of comparative physiology and pathology of the higher nervous activity. *Sbornik Voprosi sravnitelnoi fiziologii i patologii vyssh. nerv. deyat.*, pp. 110-118. Leningrad: Medgiz.

Bastian, H. C. (1869). On the various forms of loss of speech in cerebral disease. *Brit. For. Med. Chir. Rev.*, *43*, 209-236, 470-492.

Basser, L. S. (1962). Hemiplegia of early onset and the faculty of speech with special reference to the effects of hemispherectomy. *Brain, 85*, 427-460.

Bates, J. A. V. (1953). Stimulation of the medial surface of the cerebral hemisphere after hemispherectomy. *Brain, 76*, 405-447.

Batini, C., Radulovacki, M., Kado, R. T. and Adey, W. R. (1967). Effect of interhemispheric transection on the EEG patterns in sleep and wakefulness in monkeys. *E.E.G. Clin-Neurophysiol.*, *22*, 101-112.

Belmont, L. and Birch, H. G. (1963). Lateral dominance and right-left awareness in normal children. *Child Devel.*, *34*, 257-270.

Benton, A. L. (1959). Right-left discrimination and finger localization. New York: Hoeber.

Benton, A. L. (1964). Developmental aphasia and brain damage. *Cortex 1(1)*, 40-52.

Benton, A. L. (1964). Contributions to aphasia before Broca. *Cortex, 1*, 314-327.

Benton, A. L. (1967). Constructional apraxia and the minor hemsiphere. *Conf. Neurol., 29*, 1-16.

Benton, A. L. and Joynt, R. J. (1959). Reaction time in unilateral cerebral disease. *Conf. Neurol., 19*, 247-256.

Benton, A. L., Meyers, R. and Polder, G. J. (1962). Some aspects of handedness. *Psychiat. Neurol. Basel, 14*, 321-337.

Berlucchi, G. (1966). E.E.G. studies of split-brain cats. *E.E.G. Clin. Neurophysiol., 20*, 348-356.

Berlucchi, G., Gazzaniga, M. S. and Rizzolatti, G. (1967). Microelectrode analysis of transfer of visual information by the corpus callosum. *Archives Italiennes de Biologie, 105*, 583-596.

Beritashvili, I. S. (1961). *Neural mechanisms of higher vertebrate behaviour.* Moscow.

Bertelson, P. (1965). Central intermittency twenty years later. Lecture delivered on May 4th, 1965 in St. John's College, Cambridge.

Bever, T. G., Kirk, R. and Lackner, J. (1968). An autonomic reflection of syntactic structure. *Neuropsychologia, 7*, 23-28.

Bicens, L. W. and Oakley, S. R. (1965). Memory trace disruption by cortical spreading depression. *Psychological Reports, 17(1)*, 175-178.

Bills, A. G. (1931). Blocking: A new principle in mental fatigue. *Amer. J. Psychol., 43*, 230-245.

Black, P. and Myers, R. E. (1964). A neurological investigation of eye-hand control in the chimpanzee. In *Functions of the corpus callosum*, ed. Ettlinger, G. London: Churchill.

Blakemore, C. and Falconer, M. A. (1967). Long-term effects of anterior temporal lobectomy on certain cognitive functions. *J. Neurol. Neurosurg. Psychiat., 30*, 364-367.

Blakemore, C. and Pettigrew, J. D. (1970). Eye dominance in the visual cortex. *Nature, 225*, 426-429.

Blyth, K. W. (1963). Ipsilateral confusion in 2 choice, 4 choice responses with the hands and the feet. *Nature, 199*, 1312.

Blyth, K. W. (1964). Errors in a 4-choice R. T. task with hands and feet. *Nature, 201*, 641.

Bocca, E., Calearo, C., Cassinari, V. and Migliavacca, F. (1955). Testing 'cortical' hearing in temporal lobe tumours. *Acta Oto-Laryngol., 45*, 289-304.

Bogen, J. E. (1969a). The other side of the brain. I; Dysgraphia and dyscopia following cerebral commissurotomy. *Bull. Los Angeles Neurol. Soc.*, *34(2)*, 73-105.

Bogen, J. E. (1969b). The other side of the brain. II: An appositional mind. *Bull. Los Angeles Neurol. Soc.*, *34(3)*, 135-162.

Bogen, J. E. and Cambell, B. (1960). Total hemispherectomy in the cat. *Surg. Forum. Proc.*, *11*, 381.

Bogen, J. E. and Cambell, B. (1962). 'Recovery of foreleg' placing after ipsilateral frontal lobectomy in the hemicerebrectomized cat. *Science*, *135*, 309-310.

Bogen, J. E., Fisher, E. D. and Vogel, P. J. (1965). Cerebral commissurotomy: A Second case report. *J. Amer. Med. Assoc.*, *194*, 1328-1329.

Bogen, J. E. and Gazzaniga, M. S. (1965). Cerebral commissurotomy in man. (Minor hemisphere dominance for certain spatial functions). *J. Neurosurg.*, *23*, 394.

Bogen, J. E. and Vogel, P. J. (1962). Cerebral commissurotomy in man: Preliminary case report. *Bull. Los Angeles Neurol. Soc.*, *27*, 169.

Bok, S. T. (1959). Histonomy of the cerebral cortex. Amsterdam: Elsevier.

Bonin, G. von (1950). Essay on the cerebral cortex. Springfield, Illinois: C. Thomas.

Boone, D. R. (1965). Laterality dominance and language. *J. Kansas Med. Soc.*, *66*, 132-135.

Bossom, J. and Hamilton, C. R. (1963). Interocular transfer of prism-altered coordinations in split-brain monkeys. *J. Comp. Physiol. Psychol.*, *56(4)*, 769-774.

Brain, W. R. (1941). Visual disorientation with special references to lesions of the right cerebral hemisphere. *Brain*, *64*, 244-272.

Brainard, R. W., Irby, T. S., Fitts, P. M. and Alluisi, E. A. (1962). Some variables influencing the rate of gain of information. *J. Exp. Psychol.*, *63*, 105-110.

Branch, C., Milner, B. and Rasmussen, T. (1964). Intracarotid sodium amytal for the lateralization of cerebral speech dominance. Observations in 123 patients. *J. Neurosurg.*, *21*, 399-405.

Brebner, J. (1968). Continuing and reversing the direction of responding movements. Some exceptions to the so-called psychological refractory period. *J. Exp. Psychology*, *78(1)*, 120-127.

Bremer, F. (1958). Physiology of the corpus callosum. *Res. Pub. Ass. Nerv. Ment. Dis.*, *36*, 424-448.

Bremer, F. and Stoupel, N. (1956). Transmission interhémisphérique des influx visuels par le corps calleux. *J. Physiol. (Paris)*, *48*, 411-414.

Bricker, P. D. (1955). Information measurement and reaction time. In *Information theory in psychology*, ed. Quastler, H. Glencoe, Illinois: The Free Press.

Broadbent, D. E. (1952a). Listening to one of two synchronous messages. *J. Exp. Psychology*, *44*, 51-55.

Broadbent, D. E. (1952b). Failures of attention in selective listening. *J. Exp. Psychol.*, *44*, 428-433.

Broadbent, D. E. (1952c). Speaking and listening simultaneously. *J. Exp. Psychol.*, *43*, 267-273.

Broadbent, D. E. (1956). Listening between and during practised auditory distractions. *Brit. J. Psychol.* *47*, 51-60.

Broadbent, D. E. (1958). *Perception and communication*. Pergamon Press.

Broadbent, D. E. and Gregory, M. (1963). Division of attention and the decision theory of signal detection. *Proc. Roy. Soc. B*, *158*, 222-231.

Broadbent, D. E. and Gregory, M. (1964). Accuracy of recognition of speech presented to the right and the left ears. *Quart. J. Exp. Psychol.*, *16*, 359-360.

Broadbent, D. E. and Gregory, M. (1967). Psychological refractory period and the length of time required to make a decision. *Proc. Roy. Soc. B*, *168*, 181-193.

Broca, P. (1865). Sur la faculté du langage articulé. *Bull. Soc. d'Anthropol. (Paris)*, vol. 6.

Brown-Séquard, C. E. (1877). Dual character of the brain. Toner Lecture. *Smithsonian Misc. Collection, 291.* Washington.

Bruce, A. (1889). On the absence of the corpus callosum in the human brain with the description of a new case. *Brain*, *12*, 171.

Bruell, J. H. and Albee, G. W. (1962). Higher intellectual functions in a patient with hemispherectomy for tumours. *J. Consult. Psychol.*, *26(1)*, 90-98.

Bryan, W. L. and Harter, N. (1897). Studies in the physiology and psychology of the telegraphic language. *Psychol. Rev.*, *4*, 27-53.

Bryan, W. L. and Harter, N. (1899). Studies on the telegraphic language: The acquisition of a hierarchy of habits. *Psychol. Rev.*, *6*, 345-375.

Bryden, M. P. (1963). Ear preference in auditory perception. *J. Exp. Psychol.*, *65*, 103-105.

Bryden, M. P. (1964). Tachistoscopic recognition and cerebral dominance. *Percept. Mot. Skills*, *19*, 686.

Bryden, M. P. (1966). Left-right differences in tachistoscopic recognition: Directional scanning or cerebral dominance. *Percept. Mot. Skills*, *23*, 1127-1134.

Bryden, M. P. and Rainey, C. A. (1963). Left-right differences in tachistoscopic recognition. *J. Exp. Psychol.*, *66*, 578-581.

Brunt, M. and Goetzinger, C. P. (1968). A study of three tests of central function with normal hearing subjects. *Cortex*, *4(3)*, 288-297.

Bucy, P. C. and Fulton, J. J. (1933). Ipsilateral representation in the motor and the premotor cortex of monkeys. *Brain*, *56*, 318.

Bureš, J. (1959). Reversible decortication and behaviour. In *Second conference on the CNS and behaviour*, ed. Brazier, M. B. A., pp. 207-248. New York: Josiah Macy Jr. Foundation.

Bureš, J. and Burešová, O. (1960). The use of Leão's spreading depression in the study of interhemispheric transfer of memory traces. *J. Comp. Physiol. Psychol.*, *53*, 558-563.

Bureš, J. and Burešová, O. (1963). Cortical spreading depression as a memory disturbing factor. *J. Comp. Physiol. Psychol.*, *56*, 268-272.

Bureš, J., Burešová, O. and Fifkova, E. (1964). Interhemispheric transfer of a passive avoidance reaction. *J. Comp. Physiol. Psychol.*, *57*, 326-330.

Bureš, J. Burešová, O., Fifková, E., Olds, J., Olds, M. J. and Travis, R. P. (1961). Spreading depression and subcortical drive centres. *Physiol. Bohemoslov.*, *10*, 321-331.

Burešová, O. and Bureš, J. (1965). Interhemispheric synthesis of memory traces. *J. Comp. Physiol. Psychol.*, *59*, 211-214.

Burešová, O., Bureš, J. and Bevan, V. (1958). A contribution to the problem of the dominant hemisphere in rats. *Physiol. Bohemoslov.*, *7*, 29-36.

Burešová, O. and Bureš, J. (1969). Can the brain be improved. *Endeavour*, *105*, 139-145.

Burešová, O., Lukaszewska, I. and Bureš, J. (1966). Interhemispheric synthesis of goal alternation and jumping escape reactions. *J. Comp. Physiol. Psychol.*, *62*, 90-94.

Burt, C. (1969). Brain and consciousness. *Bull. Brit. Psychol. Soc.*, *22*, 29-36.

Busnel, R. G. (1968). Acoustic communication. In *Animal communication*, ed. Sebeok, T. A. Indiana University Press.

Butler, S. and Norrsell, U. (1968). Vocalization possibly initiated by the minor hemisphere. *Nature, 220*, 793.

Cameron, J. L. and Nicholls, A. (1921). Two rare abnormalities occurring in the same subject. Partial absence of the corpus callosum, the stomach situated entirely within the thorax. *Canad. M.A.J., 11*, 448.

Carmichael, A. E. (1966). The current status of hemispherectomy for infantile hemiplegia. *Clin. Proc. Child. Hosp. D.C. 22*: 285-293.

Carter, D. B. (1953). A further demonstration of phi-movement cerebral dominance. *J. Psychol., 36*, 299-309.

Cass, A. B. and Reeves, D. L. (1939). Partial agenesis; diagnosed by ventriculographic examination. *Arch. Surg., 39*, 667.

Černacek, J. and Podivinský, F. (1967). Late somatosensory cortical response and cerebral dominance. *Physiologia Bohemoslov., 16(3)*, 256-263.

Chadwick, J. and Mann, W. N. (1950). The medical works of Hippocrates. Oxford: Blackwell Scientific Publications.

Chang, Hs-T. (1953a). Cortical response to activity of callosal neurones. *J. Neurophysiol., 16*, 117-131.

Chang, Hs-T. (1953b). Interaction of evoked cortical potentials. *J. Neurophysiol., 16*, 133-144.

Cherry, C. (1953). Some experiments on the recognition of speech with one and two ears. *J. Acoust. Soc. Amer., 25*, 975-979.

Chomsky, N. (1964). Formal discussion. In *The acquisition of language*, eds. Bellugi, U. and Brown, R. *Monograph of the Soc. for research in child dev.*, vol. 29, No. 1.

Claes, E. (1939). Contribution à l'étude physiologique de la fonction visuelle, analyse oscillographique de l'activité spontanée et sensorielle de l'aime visuelle corticale chez le chat non anesthésié. *Arch. Int. Physiol., 48*, 181-237.

Cofoid, D. A. (1965). Interhemispheric spread and graded response in spreading cortical depression. *Psychonomic Science, 2(11)*, 343-344.

Cohen, A. I. (1966). Hand preference and developmental status of infants. *J. Genet. Psychol., 108*, 337-345.

Cohen, L. (1959). Perception of reversible figures after brain injury. *Arch. Neurol. Psychiat., 81*, 765-775.

Cole, J. (1955). Paw preference in cats related to hand preferences in animals and men. *J. Comp. Physiol. Psychol., 48*, 137-140.

Cole, M. and Zangwill, O. L. (1963). Déjà vu in temporal lobe epilepsy. *J. Neurol. Neurosurg. Psychiat., 26*, 37-38.

Collins, R. L. (1968). On the inheritance of handedness. I: laterality in inbred mice. *J. Hered., 59*, 9-12.

Cordeau, J. P. and Mancia, M. (1958). Effect of unilateral chronic lesions of the midbrain on the electrocortical activity of the cat. *Arch. Ital. Biol., 96*, 374-399.

Costa, L. D. and Vaughan, H. G. (1962). Performance of patients with lateralized cerebral lesions. *I: Verbal and perceptual tests.* J. Nerv. Ment. Diseas., 134, 162-168.

Cozzi, M. (1963). L'agenesia del corpo calloso: presentazione di un caso. *Lattante, 34*, 566-581.

Craik, K. J. W. (1948). Theory of the human operator in control systems. II: Man as an element in a control system. *Brit. J. Psychol., 38*, 142-148.

Cress, R. H., Taylor, L. S., Allen, B. G. and Holden, R. W. (1963). Normal motor nerve conduction velocities in the upper extremities and their relation to handedness. *Arch. Phys. Med., 44*, 216-219.

Critchley, M. (1953). *The parietal lobes.* London: Arnold.

Critchley, M. (1961). Broca's contribution to aphasia reviewed a century later. In *Scientific aspects of neurology*. ed. Garland, H. Baltimore: Williams and Wilkins.

Critchley, M. (1962). Speech and speech loss in relation to the quality of the brain. In *Interhemispheric relations and cerebral dominance*. Baltimore: Johns Hopkins Press.

Critchley, M. (1970). Asphasiology and other aspects of language. London: Edward Arnold.

Cronholm, J., Grodsky, M. and Behar I. (1963). Situational factors in the lateral preference of rhesus monkeys. *J. Genet. Psychol., 103*, 167-174.

Crossman, E. R. F. W. (1953). Entropy and choice time: the effect of frequency unbalance on choice response. *Quart. J. Exp. Psychol., 5*, 41-51.

Crossman, E. R. F. W. (1956). The information capacity of the human operator in symbolic and non-symbolic control processes. In *The application of information theory to human operator problems*, ed. Draper, J. W.R.(D) No. 2/56. Ministry of Supply, Gt. Britain.

Curtis, H. J. (1940a). Intercortical connections of the corpus callosum as indicated by evoked potentials. *J. Neurophysiol., 3*, 407-413.

Curtis, H. J. (1940b). An analysis of cortical potentials mediated by the corpus callosum. *J. Neurophysiol., 3*, 414-422.

Curtis, H. J. and Bard, P. (1939). Intercortical connections of the corpus callosum as indicated by evoked potentials. *Am. J. Physiol., 126*, 473.

Davis, R. (1956). The limits of the psychological refractory period. *Quart. J. Exp. Psychol., 8*, 24-38.

Davis, R., Moray, N. and Treisman, Anne (1961). Imitative responses and the rate of gain of information. *Quart. J. Exp. Psychol., 13*, 78-89.

Dandy, W. E. (1928). Removal of right cerebral hemisphere for certain tumours with hemiplegia. *J. Amer. Med. Ass., 90*, 823-825.

Dandy, W. E. (1933). Physiological studies following extirpation of the right cerebral hemisphere in man. *Johns Hopk. Hosp. Bull., 53*, 31-51.

Dandy, W. E. (1936). Operative experiences in cases of pineal tumours. *Arch. Surg., 33*, 19.

Davidoff, L. M. and Dyke, C. G. (1934). Agenesis of the corpus callosum. *Amer. J. Röent., 32*, 1-10.

Dearborn, W. F. (1933). Structural factors which condition special disability in reading. *Proc. Amer. Ass. Ment. Defic., 38*, 266-284.

Delisle Burns B. (1958). *The mammalian cerebral cortex.* London: Edward Arnold.

Delprato, D. J. (1965). Note on the effect of cortical spreading depression on open-field behaviour. *Psychological Reports, 17(3)*, 714-722.

DeLucchi, M. R., Garoutte, B. and Aird, R. T. (1961). Lack of effect of mid-sagittal section through corpus callosum and massa intermedia on bilateral synchrony of the EEG of the cat. *Electronenceph. Clin. Neurophysiol., 13*, 306-307.

Dethier, V. G. and Stellar, E. (1961). Animal behaviour: its evolutionary and neurological basis. Englewood Cliffs, N.J.: Prentice-Hall.

Diamond, I. T. and Hall, W. C. (1969). Evolution of neocortex. *Science, 164*, 251-262.

Diamond, I. T. (1967). The sensory neocortex. *Contrib. Sens. Physiol., 2*, 1-49.

Dide, M. (1938). Les désorientations temporo-spatiales et la prépondérance de l'hémisphère droit dans les agnoso-akinésis proprioceptives. *Encephale, 2*, 276-294.

Dimond, S. J. (1963). Anticipatory behaviour and the timing of skilled performance. Ph.D. thesis, University of Bristol Library.

Dimond, S. J. (1966). Facilitation through the use of the timing system. *J. Exp. Psychol.*, 71, 181-183.

Dimond, S. J. (1968). Response competition between the hands. Talk delivered to the British Psychological Society, April 1968.

Dimond, S. J. (1969a). The hemispheric control of Reaction Time. Talk delivered to the Experimental Psychological Society, January 1969.

Dimond, S. J. (1969b). Hemisphere function and immediate memory. *Psychonomic Science*, 16, 111-112.

Dimond, S. J. (1970a). The refractoriness of the cerebral hemispheres on language and reaction time tasks. *Bull. Brit. Psychol. Soc.*, 23, No. 79, 140.

Dimond, S. J. (1970b). Cerebral dominance or lateral preference in motor control. *Acta Psychol.*, 31, 196-198.

Dimond, S. J. (1970c). Hemisphere refractoriness and the control of reaction time. *Quart. J. Exp. Psychol.*, 24, 610-617.

Dimond, S. J. (1970d). Response competition between the hands. *Quart. J. Exp. Psychol.*, 22, 513-520.

Dimond, S. J. (1970e). *The social behaviour of animals*. London: Batsford.

Dimond, S. J. (1971a). Hemisphere function and word registration. *J. Exp. Psychol.* 87, 183-186.

Dimond, S. J. (1971b). A reappraisal of the concept of cerebral dominance. *J. of Motor Behaviour 3*, 57-62.

Dimond, S. J. and Beaumont, G. (1971). The use of two cerebral hemispheres to increase brain capacity. *Nature 232*, 270-271.

Downer, J. L. de C. (1959). Changes in visually guided behaviour following mid sagittal division of optic chiasma and corpus callosum in monkeys (*Macaca mulatta*). *Brain, 82*, 251-259.

Dreifuss, F. E. (1963). Delayed development of hemispheric dominance. *Arch. Neurol. Chicago, 8(5)*, 510-514.

Eason, G., Groves, P., White, C. T. and Oden, D. (1967). Evoked cortical potentials: Relation to visual field and handedness. *Science, 156 (3782)*, 1643-1646.

Eccles, J. (1965). The brain and the unity of conscious experience. The 19th Arthur Stanley Eddington Memorial Lecture. Cambridge, England: University Printing House.

Edwards, E. (1964). *Information transmission: an introductory guide to the application of the theory of information to the human species*. Chapman and Hall.

Efron, R. (1963). The effect of handedness on the perception of simultaneity and temporal order. *Brain, 86*, 261-284.

Egan, J. P., Carterette, E. C. and Thwing, E. J. (1954). Some factors affecting multi-channel listening. *J. Acoust. Soc. Amer., 26*, 774-782.

Eisenson, J. (1962). Language and intellectual modifications associated with right cerebral damage. *Language and Speech, 5(2)*, 49-53.

Elithorn, A. and Barnett, T. J. (1967). Apparent individual differences in channel capacity. *Acta Psychol., 27*, 75-83.

Erickson, T. C. (1940). Spread of the epileptic discharge: an experimental study of the after discharge induced by electrical stimulation of the cerebral cortex. *Arch. Neurol. Psychiat. (Chic.), 43*, 429-452.

Ertl, J. and Schafer, E. W. P. (1967). Cortical activity preceding speech. *Life Sciences, 6*, 473-479.

Ettlinger, G. (1961). Lateral preferences in monkeys. *Behaviour, 17,* 275-287.

Ettlinger, G. (1964). Lateral preferences in the monkey. *Nature, 204,* 606.

Ettlinger, G., Jackson, C. V. and Zangwill, O. L. (1955). Dysphasia following right temporal lobectomy in a right-handed man. *J. Neurol. Neurosurg. Psychiat., 18,* 214-217.

Ettlinger, G. and Morton, H. B. (1963). Callosal section: its effect on performance of a bimanual skill. *Science, 139,* 485-486.

Falconer, M. A. (1960). The treatment of encephalotrigeminal angiomatosis (Sturge-Weber Disease) by hemispherectomy. *J. Neurol. Psychiat., 23,* 81.

Falek, A. (1959). Handedness, a family study. *Amer. J. Hum. Genet., 11,* 52-62.

Ferguson, G. A. (1954). On learning and human ability. *Canad. J. Psychol., 8,* 95-112.

Ferguson, G. A. (1956). On transfer and the abilities of man. *Canad. J. Psychol., 10,* 121-131.

Feld, M. (1957). Indications et résultats des hémisphérectomies. *Rev. Neuropsychiat. Infant. Hyg. Ment. Enfance Paris, 5,* 674-676.

Ferrier, D. (1886). *The functions of the brain.* 2nd edition. New York: G. P. Putnam's Sons.

Foerster, O. (1936). *Motorische Felder und Bahnen. Handbuch der Neurologie,* eds. Bumke, O. and Foerster, O. vol. 6, pp. 1-357. Berlin: Julius Springer.

Forgays, D. G. (1953). The development of differential word recognition. *J. Exp. Psychol., 45,* 165-168.

Fielding, U. (1968). The earliest mammalian brains in the Hunterian Museum in the light of recent interpretation of cerebral structure. *Ann. Roy. Coll. Surg. Eng., 42,* 114-123.

Filimonoff, I. N. (1964). Homologies of the cerebral formations of mammals and reptiles. *J. für Hirnforschung, 7,* 229-251.

Finch, G. (1941). Chimpanzee handedness. *Science, 94,* 117-118.

French, L. A. and Johnson, D. R. (1955a). Observations on the motor system following cerebral hemispherectomy. *Neurology, 5,* 11-14.

French, L. A. and Johnson, D. R. (1955b). Examination of sensory systems in patients after hemispherectomy. *Neurology, 5,* 390-393.

French, L. A., Johnson, D. R., Brown, I. A. and Van Bergen, F. B. (1955). Hemispherectomy for control of intractable convulsive seizures. *J. Neurosurg., 12,* 154-164.

French, L. A. *et al.* (1966). Hemispherectomy, its influence on sensory perception and function of the upper extremity. *Clin. Orthop., 46,* 83-86.

Fritsch, G. and Hitzig, E. (1870). Ueber die elektrische Erregbarkeit des Grosshirns. *Arch. Anat. Physiol. wiss. Med., 37,* 300-332.

Gardner, W. J., Karnosh, L. J., McClure, Jr., C. C. and Gardner, A. K. (1955). Residual function following hemispherectomy for tumour and for infantile hemiplegia. *Brain, 78,* 487-502.

Garner, W. R. (1969). Speed of discrimination with redundant stimulus attributes. *Perception and Psychophysics, 6(4),* 221-224.

Garoutte, B., Aird, R. B. and Diamond, M. C. (1961). The electroencephalographic pacemaker and function of the corpus callosum. *Trans. Amer. Neurol. Ass., 86,* 153-156.

Gazzaniga, M. S. (1965). Some effects of cerebral commissurotomy on monkey and man. *Diss. Abstracts, 26(1),* 501-502.

Gazzaniga, M. S. (1966a). Interhemispheric cueing systems remaining after section of neocortical commissures in monkeys. *Exp. Neurol., 16(1),* 28-35.

Gazzaniga, M. S. (1966b). Visuomotor integration in split brain monkeys with other cerebral lesions. *Exp. Neurol., 16,* 289-298.

Gazzaniga, M. S. (1968). Short term memory and brain-bisected man. *Psychonomic Science*, *12(5)*, 161-162.

Gazzaniga, M. S. (1969). Cross-cueing mechanisms and ipsilateral eye-hand control in split-brain monkeys. *Exp. Neurol.*, *23*, 11-17.

Gazzaniga, M. S. (1970a). Personal communication.

Gazzaniga, M. S. (1970b). *The bisected brain*. New York: Appleton-Century-Crofts.

Gazzaniga, M. S., Bogen, J. E. and Sperry, R. W. (1965). Observations on visual perception after disconnection of the cerebral hemispheres in man. *Brain*, *8*, 221-236.

Gazzaniga, M. S., Berlucchi, G. and Rizzolatti, G. (1967). Physiological mechanisms underlying transfer of visual learning in corpus callosum of cat. *Fed. Proc. Fed. Am. Socs. Exp. Biol. 26*, 590.

Gazzaniga, M. S., Bogen, J. E. and Sperry, R. W. (1963). Laterality effects in somesthesis following cerebral commissurotomy in man. *Neuropsychologia*, *1*, 209-215.

Gazzaniga, M. S., Bogen, J. E. and Sperry, R. W. (1967). Dyspraxia following division of the cerebral commissures. *Arch. Neurol. (Chic.)*, *12*, 606-612.

Gazzaniga, M. S. and Sperry, R. W. (1966). Simultaneous double discrimination response following brain bisection. *Psychonomic Science*, *4(7)*, 261-262.

Gazzaniga, M. S. and Sperry, R. W. (1967). Language after section of the cerebral commissures. *Brain*, *90*, 131-148.

Gazzaniga, M. S. and Young, E. D. (1967). Effects of commissurotomy on the processing of increasing visual information. *Experimental Brain Research*, *3*, 368-371.

Gesell, A. and Ames, L. B. (1947). The development of handedness. *J. Genet. Psychol.*, *70*, 155-175.

Gerstmann, J. (1927). Fineragnosie und isolierte Agraphie: ein neues Syndrom. *Zeitschr. Neurol. Psychiat.*, *108*, 152-177.

Geschwind, N. (1965). Disconnexion syndromes in animals and man. *Brain*, *88*, II, 237-294 (1st Part), 585-644 (2nd Part).

Geschwind, N. (1965). The problem of language in relation to the phylogenetic development of the brain. *Sist. Nerv.*, *17*, 411-419.

Geschwind, N. (1967). The neural basis of language. In *Research in verbal behaviour and some neurophysiological implications*. New York: Academic Press.

Geschwind, N. (1970). Aphasias and related disturbances. In *Textbook of medicine*, ed. Wilkins, R. W. Boston: Little, Brown and Co.

Geschwind, N. and Kaplan, E. (1962a). Human split-brain syndromes. *New. Engl. J. Med.*, *266*, 1013.

Geschwind, N. and Kaplan, E. (1962b). A human cerebral disconnection syndrome. *Neurology*, *12(10)*, 675-685.

Geschwind, N. and Levitsky, W. (1968). Human Brain: Left-right asymmetries in temporal speech region. *Science*, *161*, 186.

Ghent, L., Semmes, J., Weinstein, S. and Teuber, H. L. (1955). Tactile discrimination after unilateral brain injury in man. *Amer. Psychologist*, *10*, 408.

Ghent, L., Weinstein, S., Semmes, J. and Teuber, H. (1955). Effect of unilateral brain injury in man on learning of a tactual discrimination. *J. Comp. Physiol.*, *48*, 478-481.

Gillies, S. M., MacSweeney, D. A. and Zangwill, O. L. (1960). A note on some unusual handedness patterns. *Quart. J. Exp. Psychol.*, *12*, 113-116.

Glickstein, M. and Sperry, R. W. (1960). Intermanual somesthetic transfer in split-brain rhesus monkeys. *J. Comp. Physiol. Psychol.*, *53*, 322-327.

Glonig, I., Glonig, K., Haub, G. and Quatember, R. (1969). Comparison of verbal behaviour in right-handed and non-right handed patients with anatomically verified lesion of one hemisphere. *Cortex*, *5(1)*, 41-52.

Goetzinger, C. and Angell, S. (1965). Audiological assessment in acoustic tumours and cortical lesions. *Eye, Ear, Nose, Throat, Mon.*, *44*, No. 6.

Goldstein, K. (1948). *Language and language disturbances*. New York: Grune and Stratton.

Goldstein, R., Goodman, A. and King, R. (1956). Hearing and speech in infantile hemiplegia before and after left hemispherectomy. *Neurology*, *6*, 869-875.

Goldstein, R. (1961). Hearing and speech in follow-up of left hemispherectomy. *J. Speech Hear. Dis.*, *26*, 126-129.

Gollander, M. and Ochs, S. (1963). Evaluation of EEG depression as an index of spreading depression in chronic preparations. *Amer. Psychologist, 18* 431.

Grafstein, B. (1956). Mechanism of spreading cortical depression. *J. Neurophysiol.*, *19*, 154-171.

Griew, S. (1958). Information gain in tasks involving different stimulus response relationships. *Nature, 182,* 1819.

Griew, S. (1959). Set to respond and the effect of interrupting signals upon tracking performance. *J. Exp. Psychol.*, *57*, 333-337.

Griew, S. (1964). Age information transmission and the positional relationship between signals and responses in the performance of a choice task. *Ergonomics, 7,* 267-277.

Griffith, H., and Davidson, M. (1966). Long term changes in intellect and behaviour after hemispherectomy. *J. Neurol. Neurosurg. Psychiat.*, *29*, 571-576.

Groden, G. (1969). Lateral preferences in normal children. *Percept. and Mot. Skills, 28(1),* 213-214.

Grogono, J. L. (1968). Children with agenesis of the corpus callosum. *Develop. Med. Child Neurol.*, *10*, 613-616.

Guyton, A. G. (1966). *Textbook of medical physiology*. Philadelphia and London: Saunders.

Gyepes, M. T. and Gannon, W. E. (1963). Agenesis of the corpus callosum. *N.Y. State J. Med.*, *63*, 1385-1387.

Haggard, M. (1970). Synthetic computer formed speech. Personal communication.

Hall, K. R. and Mayer, B. (1966). Hand preference and dexterities of captive patas monkeys. *Folia Primat. (Basel), 4,* 169-185.

Hamilton, C. R. (1967). Effects of brain bisection on eye-hand coordination in monkeys wearing prisms. *J. Comp. Physiol. Psychol.*, *64*, 434-443.

Hamilton, C. R., Hillyard, S. A. and Sperry, R. W. (1968). Interhemispheric comparison of colour in split-brain monkeys. *Exp. Neurol.*, *21*, 486-494.

Harcum, E. R. and Jones, M. L. (1962). Letter recognition within words flashed left and right of fixation. *Science, 138,* 444-445.

Harcum, E. R. and Finkel, M. E. (1963). Explanation of Mishkin and Forgays result as a directional reading conflict. *Canad. J. Psychol.*, *17*, 224-234.

Harreveld, A. von. (1958). Changes in the diameter of apical dendrites during spreading depression. *Amer. J. Physiol.*, *192*, 457-463.

Harreveld, A. von. (1959). Compounds in brain extracts causing spreading depression of cerebral cortical activity and contraction of crustacean muscle. *J. Neurochem.*, *3*, 300-315.

Harreveld, A. von. (1966). *Brain tissue electrolytes*. London and Washington, D.C.: Butterworths.

Harreveld, A. von, Terres, G., and Dernburg, E. A. (1956). Cortical discontinuity and propagation of spreading depression. *Amer. J. Physiol., 184*, 233-238.

Harreveld, A. von, and Stamm, J. S. (1952). Vascular concomitants of spreading cortical depression. *J. Neurophysiol., 15*, 487-496.

Harreveld, A. von, Stamm, J. S. and Christensen, E. (1956). Spreading depression in rabbit, cat and monkey. *Amer. J. Physiol., 184*, 312-320.

Head, H. (1926). *Aphasia and kindred disorders of speech.* Cambridge University Press.

Hebb, D. O. (1939). Intelligence in man after large removals of cerebral tissue defects following right temporal lobectomy. *J. Gen. Psychol., 21*, 437-446.

Hebb, D. O. (1959). Intelligence, brain function and the theory of mind. *Brain, 82*, 260-275.

Hécaen, H. (1959). Dominance hémisphérique et préférence manuelle. *Evol. Psychiat., 1*, 1-50.

Hécaen, H. (1962). Clinical symptomatology in right and left hemispheric lesions. In *Interhemispheric relations and cerebral dominance*, ed. Mountcastle, V. B. Baltimore: Johns Hopkins Press.

Hécaen, H. and Badaracco, G. (1956). Séméiologie des hallucinations visuelles en clinique neurologique. *Acta Neurol. Latinoam., 2*, 23-58.

Hécaen, H. and Ajuriaguerra, J. (1964). *Left Handedness.* New York: Grune and Stratton.

Henschen, S. E. (1926). On the function of the right hemisphere of the brain in relation to the left in speech, music and calculation. *Brain, 49*, 110-123.

Heron, W. (1957). Perception as a function of retinal locus and attention. *Amer. J. Psychol., 70*, 38-48.

Hick, W. E. (1952). On the rate of gain of information. *Quart. J. Exp. Psychol., 4*, 11-26.

Hildreth, G. (1949a). The development and training of hand dominance. *Part I: J. Genet. Psychol., 75*, 197-220.

Hildreth, G. (1949b). The development and training of hand dominance. II. Developmental tendencies in handedness. *J. Genet. Psychol., 75*, 221-254.

Hillier, W. F. (1954). Hemispherectomy for malignant glioma. *Neurology, 4*, 718-721.

Hinde, R. (1966). *Animal behaviour.* New York: McGraw-Hill.

Hirata, K. I. and Osaka, R. (1967). Tachistoscopic recognition of Japanese materials in left and right visual fields. *Psychologia, 10*, 7-18.

Hirsh, I. J. (1950). The relation between localization and intelligibility. *J. Acoust. Soc. Amer., 22*, 196-200.

Hodgson, W. R. (1967). Audiological report of a patient with left hemispherectomy. *J. Speech, Hear. Dis., 32(1)*, 39-45.

Holloway, R. L. Jr. (1968). The evolution of the primate brain: some aspects of quantitative relations. *Brain Res., 7*, 121-172.

Hubel, D. H. (1967). Cortical and callosal connections concerned with the vertical meridian of visual fields in the cat. *J. Neurophysiol., 30*, 1561-1573.

Hyndman, O. R. and Penfield, W. (1937). Agenesis of the corpus callosum. *Arch. Neurol. Psychiat. (Chic.), 37*, 1251.

Inglis, J. (1965). Dichotic listening and cerebral dominance. *Acta Otolaryngol., 60*, 231-237.

Jackson, J. H. (1874). On the duality of the brain. *Med. Press 1*, 19. Reprinted in *Selected writings of John Hughlings Jackson*, ed. Taylor, J. Vol. II, pp. 129-145 (1932). London: Hodder and Stoughton.

Jackson, J. H. (1876). Case of large cerebral tumour without optic neuritis and with left hemiplegia and imperception. *R. Lond. opthal. Hosp. Rep., 8,* 434.

James, W. E., Mefferd, R. B. Jr. and Wieland, B. A. (1967). Repetitive psychometric measures. Handedness and performance. *Percept. Motor Skills, 25,* 209-212.

Jankowska, E. and Gorska, T. (1960). The effects of unilateral ablations, of sensorimotor cortex on Type II conditioned reflexes in cats. I. Natural Conditioned reflexes. *Acta Biol. Exp. Warsaw, 20,* 193-209.

Jeeves, M. A. (1965). Agenesis of the corpus callosum: physiopathological and clinical aspects. *Proc. Aust. Ass. Neurol., 3,* 41-48.

Jones, D., Benton, A. L. and MacQueen, J. C. (1967). Hand preference and manipulative dexterity in normal and retarded children. *J. Ment. Defic. Res., 11,* 49-53.

Joynt, R. (1964). Paul Pierra Broca: his contribution to the knowledge of aphasia. *Cortex, 1,* 206-213.

Kaas, J., Alexrod, S. and Diamond, I. T. (1967). An ablation study of the auditory cortex in the cat using binaural tone patterns. *J. Neurophysiol., 30,* 710.

Kaplan, E., Geschwind, N. and Goodglass, H. (1961). A human split brain syndrome. *Proc. Ann. V. A. Med. Res. Conf., 12,* 38.

Kellogg, W. N. (1948). Conditioning involving the two body sides after hemi-decortication. *Amer. Psychologist, 3,* 237.

Kellogg, W. N. (1949). Locomotor and other disturbances following hemi-decortication in the dog. *J. Comp. Physiol. Psychol., 42,* 506-516.

Kennard, M. A. and Watts, J. W. (1934). The effect of section of the corpus callosum on the motor performance of monkeys. *J. Nerv. Ment. Dis., 79,* 159.

Kimura, D. (1961a). Cerebral dominance and the perception of verbal stimuli. *Canad. J. Psychol., 13,* 166-171.

Kimura, D. (1961b). Some effects of temporal-lobe damage on auditory perception. *Canad. J. Psychol., 15,* 156-165.

Kimura, D. (1962). Perceptual and memory functions of the left temporal lobe: A reply to Dr. Inglis. *Canad. J. Psychol., 16(1),* 18-22.

Kimura, D. (1963a). A note on cerebral dominance in hearing. *Acta Oto-laryngol., 56,* 617-618.

Kimura, D. (1963b). Speech lateralization in young children as determined by an auditory test. *J. Comp. Physiol. Psychol., 56,* 899-902.

Kimura, D. (1964). Left-right differences in the perception of melodies. *Quart. J. Exp. Psychol., 16,* 355-358.

Kimura, D. (1966). Dual functional assymetry of the brain in visual perception. *Neuropsychologia, 4,* 275-285.

Kimura, D. (1967). Functional asymmetry of the brain in dichotic listening. *Cortex, 3,* 163-178.

Kimura, D. (1969). Spatial localization in left and right visual fields. *Canad. J. Psychol., 23,* 445-458.

Kimura, D. (1970). Talk given to the International Neuropsychological Symposium. Cambridge.

Kimura, D. and Folb, S. (1968). Neural processing of backwards speech sounds. *Science, 161,* 395-396.

Kimura, D. and Vanderwolf, I. (1971). The relation between hand preference and the performance of individual finger movements by left and right hands. *Brain* (in press).

Knott, J. R., Ingram, W. R. and Chiles, W. D. (1955). Effects of subcortical lesions on cortical electroencephalogram in cats. *Arch. Neurol. Psychiat. (Chic.), 73,* 203-215.

Koch, F. P. and Doyle, P. J. (1957). Agenesis of the corpus callosum: report of eight cases in infancy. *J. Paed.*, *50*, 345-351.

Kohn, B. (1967). Spreading depression and stimulus control of interhemispheric transfer. *Neuropsychologia, 5(1)*, 275-286.

Kohn, B. and Myers, R. (1969). Visual information and intermanual transfer of latch-box problem solving in monkeys with commissures sectioned. *Exp. Neurol.*, *23*, 303-309.

Koppman, J. W. (1963). Effect of unilateral spreading cortical depression and task difficulty on interhemispheric transfer of avoidance learning. Unpublished doctoral dissertation. University of Illinois.

Koppman, J. W. and O'Kelly, L. I. (1966). Unilateral cortical spreading depression. A determiner of behaviour at a choice point. *J. Comp. Physiol. Psychol.*, *62*, 237-242.

Kounin, J. S. (1938). Laterality in monkeys. *J. Genet. Psychol.*, *52*, 375-393.

Kreindler, A., Fradis, A. and Sevastopol, N. (1966). Le répartition des dominances hémisphériques. *Neuropsychologia, 4*, 143-149.

Kruper, D. C., Boyle, B., and Patton, R. (1967). Eye preference in hemicerebrectomized monkeys. *Psychonomic Science, 7(3)*, 105-106.

Kruper, D. C., Patton, R. A. and Koskoff, Y. D. (1965). Position response preference following unilateral brain ablation in monkeys. *Psychonomic Science, 3*, 195-196.

Krynauw, R. A. (1950a). Infantile hemiplegia treated by removal of one cerebral hemisphere. *S. Afr. Med. Journal, 24*, 539-54.

Krynauw, R. A. (1950b). Infantile hemiplegia treated by removing one cerebral hemisphere. *J. Neurol. Neurosurg. Psychiat.*, *13*, 243-267.

Knight, A. A. (1967). Laboratory studies of response and movement times in simple repetitive tasks. Ph.D. thesis, University of Birmingham.

Knox, C. and Kimura, D. (1970). Cerebral processing of non-verbal sounds in boys and girls. *Neuropsychologia* (in press).

Kukleta, M. (1966). Application de la dépression envahissante à l'étude de la localization des traces de mémoire. *Physiology and Behaviour, 1(3)*, 229-232.

Kupferman, I. (1965). Failure of spreading depression to produce retrograde amnesia. *Psychonomic Science, 3*, 43-44.

Kupfermann, I. (1966). Is the retrograde amnesia that follows cortical spreading depression due to subcortical spread? *J. Comp. Physiol. Psychol.*, *61(3)* 466-467.

Laget, P. and de Neverlée, H. (1963). Etude du potentiel stable et de la dépression envahissante chez le lapin en cours de développement. *J. de Physiologie, 55*, 278-279.

Lange, J. (1936). Agnosien und Apraxien. Handbuch der Neurologie, eds. Bumke, O. and Foerster, O. Vol. VI, pp. 807-960. Berlin: Springer.

Landsell, H. C. (1961). Two selective deficits found to be lateralized in temporal neurosurgery patients. Paper read at 32nd annual meeting of Eastern Psychological Association, Philadelphia.

Landsell, H. (1962). Laterality of verbal intelligence in the brain. *Science, 135*, 922-923.

Larsson, K. (1962). Spreading cortical depression and the mating behaviour in male and female rats. *Z. Tierpsychol., 19*, 321-331.

Lashley, K. S. (1951). The problem of serial order in behaviour. In *Cerebral mechanisms in behaviour*. ed. Jeffress, L. A. New York: Wiley.

Lawson, E. A. (1966). Decisions concerning the rejected channel. *Quart. J. Exp. Psychol.*, *18*, 260-265.

Leaõ, A. A. P. (1944). Spreading depression of activity in the cerebral cortex. *J. Neurophysiol., 7,* 359-390.

Leaõ, A. A. P. (1947). Further observations on the spreading depression of activity in cerebral cortex. *J. Neurophysiol., 10,* 409-414.

Leaõ, A. A. P. and Morison, R. S. (1945). Propagation of spreading cortical depression. *J. Neurophysiol., 4,* 438-455.

Lee-Teng, E. and Sperry, R. W. (1966). Intermanual stereognostic size discrimination in split-brain monkeys. *J. Comp. Physiol. Psychol., 62(1),* 84-89.

Lenneberg, E. H. (1967). *Biological foundations of language.* New York: Wiley.

Leonard, J. A. (1959). Tactual choice reactions. I. *Quart. J. Exp. Psychol. 11,* 76-83.

Levy-Agresti, J. (1968). Ipsilateral projection systems and minor hemisphere function in man after neocommissurotomy. *Anat. Rec., 160,* 384.

Levy, J. (1969). Possible basis for the evolution of lateral specialization of the human brain. *Nature, 224,* 614.

Levy-Agresti, J. and Sperry, R. W. (1968). Differential perceptual capacities in major and minor hemispheres. *Proc. U.S. Nat. Acad. Sci., 61,* 1151.

Liberman, A. M. (1957). Some results of research in speech perception. *J. Acoust. Soc. Amer., 29,* 117-123.

Liberman, A. M., Cooper, F. S., Harris, K. S. and MacNeilage, P. F. (1963). A motor theory of speech perception. In *Proceedings of the speech communication seminar.* Stockholm: Royal Institute of Technology.

Liberman, A. M. *et al.* (1967). Perception of the speech code. *Psychol. Rev., 74,* 431-461.

Liberson, W. T. (1956). Experiment concerning reciprocal inhibition of antagonists elicited by electrical stimulation of agonists in a normal individual. *Amer. J. Phys. Med., 44,* 306-308.

Licklider, J. C. R. (1948). The influence of interaural phase relations upon the masking of speech by white noise. *J. Acoust. Soc. Amer., 20,* 150-159.

Liddell, E. G. T. (1955). Brain and muscle. *Proc. Brit. Assoc. Adv. Sci., 11,* 363.

Liepmann, H. (1900). Das Krankheitsbild der Apraxia (motorischen Asymbolie). *Mschr. Psychiat. Neurol., 8,* 15-44, 102-132, 182-197.

Liepmann, H. and Maas, O. (1907). Fall von linksseitiger Agraphie und Apraxie bei rechtsseitiger Lähmung. *J. Psychol. u. Neurol., 10,* 214-227.

Lobanova, L. V. (1966). Prostranstvennyĭ analiz u sobak lishënnykh kory odnogo polushariya golovnogo mozga. *Vaprosy Sravitnel'noĭ Fiziologii Analizatorov, 2,* 112-127.

Loeser, J. D. and Alvard, E. C., Jr. (1968). Agenesis of the corpus callosum. *Brain, 91,* 553-570.

Luria, A. R. (1963). *Restoration of function after brain injury.* Oxford: Pergamon Press.

Luria, A. R. (1966). *Higher cortical functions in man.* Trans. Basil Haigh. N.Y.C. Basic Books.

MacKay, H. J. (1952). Hemispherectomy in hemispastics. *Northwest Med., 51,* 363.

Mackworth, N. H. (1950). Researches in the measurement of human performance. M.R.C. Special Report Series No. 268, H. M. Stationery Office.

MacNeilage, P. F. (1970). Motor control of serial ordering of speech. *Psych. Rev., 77,* No. 3, 182-196.

Magni, F., Melzack, R. and Smith, L. J. (1960). A stereotaxic method for sectioning the corpus callosum of the cat. *Electroenceph. Clin. Neurophysiol., 12,* 517-518.

Marcie, P., Hécaen, H., Dubois, J. and Angelergues, R. (1965). Les réalisation du langage chez les malades atteints de lésions de l'hémisphere droit. *Neuropsychologia*, 3, 217-245.

Marshall, W. H. (1959). Spreading cortical depression of Leaõ. *Physiol. Rev.*, 39, 239-279.

Marshall, W. H. and Essig, C. F. (1951). Relation of air exposure of cortex to spreading depression of Leaõ. *J. Neurophysiol.*, 14, 265-273.

Marshall, W. H., Hanna, C., and Barnard, G. (1950). Relation of dehydration of the brain to certain abnormal phenomena of the cortex. *Electroenceph. Clin. Neurophysiol.*, 2, 177-185.

Marshall, C. and Walker, A. E. (1950). The electroencephalographic changes after hemispherectomy in man. *Electroenceph. Clin. Neurophysiol.*, 2, 147-156.

Mark, R. F. and Sperry, R. W. (1968). Binaural coordination in monkeys. *Experimental Neurology*, 21(1), 92-104.

McCulloch, W. S. and Garol, H. W. (1941). Cortical origin and distribution of corpus callosum and anterior commissure in the monkey *(Macaca mulatta)*. *J. Neurophysiol.*, 4, 555-563.

McFie, J. (1961). The effects of hemispherectomy on intellectual functioning in cases of infantile hemiplegia. *J. Neurol. Neurosurg. Psychiat.*, 24, 240-249.

McFie, J., Piercy, M. F. and Zangwill, O. L. (1950). Visual spatial agnosia associated with lesions of the right cerebral hemisphere. *Brain*, 73, 167-190.

McFie, J. and Zangwill, O. L. (1960). Visual-constructive disabilities associated with lesions of the left cerebral hemisphere. *Brain*, 83, 243-260.

Mehlman, A. (1969). Ear asymmetry as a function of delayed stimulus presentation. *Proc. of the 77th Annual Convention of the A.P.A.*, 4(1), 209-210.

Mello, N. K. (1965a). Interhemispheric reversal of mirror-image oblique lines after monocular training in pigeons. *Science*, 148, 252.

Mello, N. K. (1965b). Mirror image reversal in pigeons. *Science*, 149, 1519.

Meikle, T. H. (1964). Failure of interocular transfer of brightness discrimination. *Nature*, 202, 1234-1244.

Meikle, T. H. and Sechzer, J. A. (1960). Interocular transfer of brightness discrimination in split-brain cats. *Science*, 132, 734-735.

Menkes, J. H., Philippart, M. and Clark, D. B. (1964). Hereditary partial agenesis of the corpus callosum. *Arch. Neurol.*, 11, 198-208.

Mensh, I. N., Schwartz, H. G., Matarazzo, R. G. and Matarazzo, J. D. (1952). Psychological functioning following cerebral hemispherectomy in man. *A.M.A. Arch. Neurol. Psychiat.*, 67, 787-796.

Meyer, V. and Yates, H. J. (1955). Intellectual changes following temporal lobectomy for psychomotor epilepsy. *J. Neurol. Neurosurg. Psychiat.*, 18, 44-52.

Meyers, B. and Stern, W. C. (1966). Effect of bilateral spreading depression and scopolamine on motor activity in rats. *Psychological Reports*, 18(1), 267-270.

Milner, A. D. (1969). Distribution of hand preferences in monkeys. *Neuropsychologia*, 7(4), 375-377.

Milner, B. (1954). Intellectual functions of the temporal lobes. *Psychol. Bull.*, 51, 44-52.

Milner, B. (1956). Psychological defects produced by temporal lobe excision. *Res. Publ. Ass. Res. Nerv. Ment. Dis.*, 36, 244-257.

Milner, B. (1960). Impairment of visual recognition and recall after right temporal lobectomy in man. Paper read at Psychonomic Society Annual Meeting, Chicago, 1960.

Milner, B. (1962). Laterality effects in audition. In. *Interhemispheric relations and cerebral dominance*, ed. Mountcastle, V. B. Baltimore: Johns Hopkins Press.

Milner, B. (1968). Disorders of memory after brain lesions in man: Preface: Material specific and generalized memory loss. *Neuropsychologia, 6(3),* 175-179.

Milner, B., Taylor, L. and Sperry, R. W. (1968). Lateralized suppression and dichotically presented digits after commissural section in man. *Science, 161* (3837), 184-185.

Mingrino, S., Sermeran, A., Ravenna, C., Benedett, A. (1969). Nocturnal E.E.G. patterns of patients following complete or partial hemispherectomy. *Electroenceph. Clin. Neurophysiol., 27,* 99.

Mishkin, M. and Forgays, D. G. (1952). Word recognition as a function of retinal locus. *J. Exp. Psychol., 43,* 43-48.

Mogenson, G. J. (1965). Effect of spreading cortical depression on avoidance responses conditioned to peripheral or central stimulation. *Electroenceph. Clin. Neurophysiol., 18,* 663-669.

Monakhov, K. K., Fifkova, E. and Bureš, J. (1962). Vertical distribution of the slow potential change of spreading depression in the cerebral cortex of the rat. *Physiol. Bohemoslov., 11,* 269-276.

Moray, N. (1959). Attention in dichotic listening: affective cues and the influence of instruction. *Quart. J. Exp. Psychol., 11,* 56-60.

Moruzzi, G. (1939). Contribution à l'électrophysiologie du cortex moteur: fac ilitation afterdischarge et épilepsie corticales. *Arch. Internat. Physiol., 49,* 33-100.

Mowbray, G. H. (1960). Choice reaction times for skilled responses. *Quart. J. Exp. Psychol., 12,* 193-202.

Mowbray, G. H. and Rhoades, M. V. (1959). On the reduction of choice reaction times with practice. *Quart. J. Exp. Psychol., 11,* 16-23.

Mueller, W. (1963). The psychopathology of congenital lack of the corpus callosum. *Psychiat. Neurol. Med. Psychol. (Lpz.), 15,* 138-144.

Muntz, W. R. A. (1961). Interocular transfer in octopus: Bilaterality of the engram. *J. Comp. Physiol. Psychol., 54,* 192-195.

Murphy, E. H. and Venables, P. H. (1970). Ear asymmetry in the threshold of fusion of two clicks: A signal detection analysis. *Quart. J. Exp. Psychol., 22,* 288-300.

Murphy, M. M. (1962). Hand preferences of 3 diagnostic groups of severely deficient males. *Percept. Mot. Skills, 14(3),* 508.

Myers, R. E. (1956). Functions of corpus callosum in interocular transfer. *Brain, 79,* 358.

Myers, R. E. (1957). Corpus callosum and interhemispheric communication: enduring memory effects, *Fed. Proc. Fed. Amer. Socs. Exp. Biol., 16,* 398.

Myers, R. E. (1959). Interhemispheric communication through the corpus callosum: Limitations under conditions of conflict. *J. Comp. Physiol. Psychol., 52,* 6-9.

Myers, R. E. (1961). Corpus callosum and visual gnosis. In *Brain mechanisms and learning.* eds. Fessard, A., Gerard, R. W., Konorski, J. and Delafresnaye, J. F. Oxford: Blackwell Scientific Publications.

Myers, R. E. (1962). Transmission of visual information within and between the hemispheres. A behavioural study. In *Interhemispheric relations and cerebral dominance.* ed. Mountcastle, V. B. Baltimore: Johns Hopkins Press.

Myers, R. E. (1964). The neocortical commissures and interhemispheric transmission of information. In *Functions of the corpus callosum.* ed. Ettlinger, G. London: J. and A. Churchill.

Myers, R. E. and Henson, C. O. (1960). Role of corpus callosum in transfer of tactuokinesthetic learning in chimpanzee. *Arch. Neurol. (Chic.), 3*, 404-409.

Nadel, L. (1966). Cortical spreading depression and habituation. *Psychonomic Science, 5(3)*, 119-120.

Naiman, J. and Fraser, F. C. (1955). Agenesis of the corpus callosum: A report of two cases in siblings. *Arch. Neurol. Psychiat., 74*, 182-185.

Newcombe, F. (1969). *Missile wounds of the brain.* Oxford Neurological Monographs. Oxford University Press.

Newcombe, F., Oldfield, C. and Wingfield, A. (1965). Object-naming by dysphasic patients. *Nature, 207*, 1217-1218.

Newcombe, F., Oldfield, R. C., Ratcliff, G. G. and Wingfield, W. (1971). The recognition and naming of object drawings by men with focal brain wounds. *J. Neurol. Neurosurg. Psychiat.* (in press).

Nielsen, J. M. (1946). Agnosia, apraxia, asphasia, their value in cerebral localization. New York: Hoeber.

Noble, J. (1966). Mirror-images and the forebrain commissures of the monkey. *Nature, 211*, 1263-1266.

Nobler, M. P., Shapiro, J. H. and Fine, D. I. M. (1963). The cerebral angiogram in agenesis of the corpus callosum. *Amer. J. Roent., 90*, 522-527.

Norman, D. A. (1969). Memory while shadowing. *Quart. J. Exp. Psychol., 21(1)*, 85-93.

Oakley, D. A. and Russell, I. S. (1968). Mass action and pavlovian conditioning. *Psychonomic Science, 12(3)*, 91-92.

Obrador, A. S. (1964). Cerebral localization and organization. Eds. Schaltenbrand, G. and Woolsey, C. W. Madison: University of Wisconsin Press.

Obrador, S. and Larramendi, M. H. (1950). Some observations on the brain rhythms after surgical removal of a cerebral hemisphere. *Electroenceph. Clin. Neurophysiol., 2*, 143-146.

Ochs, S. (1962). The nature of spreading depression in neural networks. *Int. Rev. Neurobiol., 4*, 1-69.

Ochs, S. (1966). Neural mechanisms of the cerebral cortex. In *Frontiers in physiological psychology*, ed. Russell, R. W. Academic Press.

Ojemann, R. H. (1930). Studies in handedness. I: A technique for testing unimanual handedness. II: Testing bimanual handedness. *J. Educ. Psychol., 21*, 597-611, 695-702.

Oldfield, R. C. (1966). Things, words and the brain. *Quart. J. Exp. Psychol., 18*, 340-353.

Oldfield, R. C. (1969). Handedness in musicians. *Brit. J. Psychol., 60*, 91-99.

Olds, J. and Travis, R. P. (1960). Spreading depression and self-stimulation. *Fed. Proc. Fed. Amer. Socs. Exp. Biol., 19*, 293.

Orbach, J. (1953). Retinal locus as a factor in recognition of visually perceived words. *Amer. J. Psychol., 65*, 555-562.

Orton, S. T. (1937). Reading, writing and speech problems in children. London: Chapman and Hall.

Osawa, K. *et al.* (1966). Long term observations of hemispherectomized dogs. *Brain Nerve (Tokyo), 18*, 805: 11.

Osson, D. (1966). Mental examination of 12 hemispherectomized patients. *Rev. Neuropsychiat. Infant., 11*, 89-98.

Oxbury, J. M. and Oxbury, S. M. (1969). Effects of temporal lobectomy on the report of dichotically presented digits. *Cortex, 5(1)*, 3-14.

Oxbury, S., Oxbury, J. and Gardiner, J. (1967). Laterality effects in dichotic listening. *Nature, 214*, 742-743.

Palmer, R. C. (1964). Development of a differentiated handedness. *Psychol. Bull., 62*, 257.

Parsons, O. A., Vega, A., Jr. and Burn, J. (1969). Different psychological effects of lateralized brain damage. *J. Consult. Clin. Psychol.*, *33(5)*, 551-557.

Paterson, A. and Zangwill, O. L. (1944). Disorders of visual space perception associated with lesions of the right cerebral hemisphere. *Brain, 67*, 331-358.

Penfield, W. (1950). The supplementary motor area in the cerebral cortex of man. *Arch. Psychiat. Nervenkr.*, *185*, 670-674.

Penfield, W. (1958). Functional localization in temporal and deep sylvian areas. *Res. Publ. Assoc. Res. Nerv. Ment. Dis.*, *36*, 210-226.

Penfield, W. (1965). Conditioning the uncommitted cortex for language. *Brain, 88*, 787-798.

Penfield, W. and Boldrey, E. (1937). Somatic motor and sensory representation in the cerebral cortex of man as studied by electrical stimulation. *Brain, 60*, 389.

Penfield, W. and Roberts, L. (1959). *Speech and brain mechanics*. New Jersey: Princeton University Press.

Peterson, G. M. and Devine, J. V. (1963). Transfers in handedness in the rat resulting from small cortical lesions after limited forced Practice. *J. Comp. Physiol. Psychol.*, *56(4)*, 752-756.

Peterson, G. M. and Gucker, D. K. (1959). Factors influencing identification of the handedness area in the cerebral cortex of the rat. *J. Comp. Physiol. Psychol.*, *52*, 279-283.

Peterson, L. R. and Kroener, S. (1964). Dichotic stimulation and retention. *J. Exp. Psychol.*, *68*, 125-130.

Pierce, J. R. and Karlin, J. E. (1957). Reading rates and the information rate of a human channel. *Bell Syst. Tech. J.*, *36*, 497-516.

Piercy, M. (1964). The effects of cerebral lesions on intellectual function: a review of current research trends. *Brit. J. Psychiat.*, *110*, 310-352.

Piercy, M. and Smyth, V. (1962). Right hemisphere dominance for certain non-verbal intellectual skills. *Br. J. Psychiat.*, *83*, 775-790.

Pöetzl, L. (1928). Die optisch-agnostischen Störungen. Leipzig: Deuticke.

Popov, N. F. (1953). Issledovaniya po fiziologii kory golovnogo mozga zhivotnykh. Moscow: Sovetskaya Nauka.

Poulton, E. C. (1953). Two-channel listening. *J. Exp. Psychol.*, *46*, 91-96.

Powell, C. A. (1962). Tachistoscopic recognition of unfamiliar visual material. Unpublished thesis, McGill University.

Pribram, K. H., Ahumada, A., Hartog, J. and Roos, L. A. (1964). A progress report on the neurological processes disturbed by frontal lesions. In *The frontal granular cortex and behaviour*. eds. Warren, J. M. and Akert, K. New York: McGraw-Hill.

Provins, K. A. (1956). Handedness and skill. *Quart. J. Exp. Psychol.*, *8*, 79-95.

Provins, K. A. (1967). Motor skills, handedness and behaviour. *Aust. J. Psychol.*, *19*, 137-150.

Provins, K. A. (1967). Handedness and motor skill. *Med. J. Aust.*, *2*, 468-470.

Putnam, S. J., Megirian, D. and Manning, J. W. (1968). Marsupial interhemispheric relation. *J. Comp. Neurol.*, *132*, 227-234.

Rabbitt, P. (1965). Response facilitation on repetition of a limb movement. *Brit. J. Psychol.*, *56*, 303-304.

Rabedeau, R. G. (1966). Retrograde amnesia due to spreading cortical depression. *Psychonomic Science, 5(3)*, 113-114.

Radulovački, M., Batini, C., Lyubimov, N. N., Rhodes, J. M., Kado, R. T. and Adey, W. R. (1965). E.E.G. sleep patterns in split-brain monkeys. *Fed. Proc. Fed. Amer. Socs. Exp. Biol.*, *24*, 339.

Ray, O. S. and Emley, G. (1964). Time factors in interhemispheric transfer of learning. *Science, 144*, 76-78.

Reeves, D. L. and Carville, C. B. (1938). Complete agenesis of corpus callosum: report of four cases. *Bull. Los Angeles Neurol. Soc., 3*, 169-181.

Riklan, M. and Diller, L. (1961). Visual motor performance before and after chemosurgery of the basal ganglia in parkinsonism. *J. Nerv. Ment. Dis., 132*, 307-313.

Roberts, D. G., Provins, K. A. and Morton, R. J. (1959). Arm strength and body dimensions. *Human Biol., 31*, 334-343.

Robinson, J. S. and Voneida, T. J. (1964). Central cross-midline integration of patterned visual inputs in split-brain cats. *Amer. Psychologist, 19*, 506.

Roone, R. N. and Williams, G. H., Jr. (1962). Diencephalic seizures accompanying agenesis of the corpus callosum. *Trans. Amer. Neurol. Ass., 87*, 237.

Rosenzweig, M. R. (1951). Representations of the two ears at the auditory cortex. *Amer. J. Physiol., 167*, 147-158.

Rosier, M. and Choppy, M. A. (1956). A propos d'une hémisphérectomie chez un adulte atteinte d'une hémiplégie cérébrale infantile avec. comitialité grave. *Neuro-chirurgie, 2*, 446-450.

Rossi, G. F., Minobe, K. and Candia, O. (1963). An experimental study of the hypnogenic mechanisms of the brain stem. *Arch. Ital. Biol., 101*, 470-492.

Rowe, S. N. (1937). Mental changes following the removal of the right cerebral hemisphere for brain tumour. *Amer. J. Psychiat., 94*, 605-614.

Rüdiger, W. and Fifková, E. (1963). Operant behaviour and subcortical drive during spreading depression. *J. Comp. Physiol. Psychol., 56*, 375-379.

Russell, I. S. and Ochs, S. (1960). Localization of behavioural control in one cortical hemisphere. *Physiologist, 3*, 152.

Russell, I. S. and Ochs, S. (1961). One-trial interhemispheric transfer of a learning engram. *Science, 133*, 1077-1078.

Russell, I. S. and Ochs, S. (1963). Localization of a memory trace in one cortical hemisphere and transfer to the other hemisphere. *Brain, 86*, 37-54.

Russell, J. R. and Reitan, R. M. (1955). Psychological abnormalities in agenesis of the corpus callosum. *J. Nerv. Ment. Dis., 121*, 205-214.

Russell, W. R. and Espir, M. L. E. (1961). Traumatic aphasia. London: Oxford University Press.

Russell, W. R. and Young, R. R. (1969). Missile wounds of the parasagittal Rolandic area. In *Recent advances in neurology.* ed. Locke, S. Boston: Little, Brown.

Rutledge, L. T. and Kennedy, T. T. (1960). Extracallosal delayed responses to cortical stimulation in chloralosed cat. *J. Neurophysiol., 23*, 188-196.

Samson, Wright. (1965). *Applied physiology.* Revised by C. A. Keele and E. Neil. Oxford Medical Publications.

Satz, P. (1968). Laterality effects in dichotic listening. *Nature, 218*, 277-278.

Satz, P., Achenback, K. and Fennell, E. (1967). Correlations between assessed manual laterality and predicted speech laterality in a normal population. *Neuropsychologia, 5(4)*, 295-310.

Saul, R. E. and Sperry, R. W. (1968). Absence of commissurotomy symptoms with agenesis of the corpus callosum. *Neurology, 18*, 307.

Schadé, J. P. (1964). Maturational changes in cerebral cortex. III: Effects of methionine sulfoximine on some electrical parameters and dendritic organization of cortical neurones. In *The developing brain,* eds. Himwhich, W. A. and Himwhich, H. E. Prog. in Brain Research. Amsterdam: Elsevier.

Schafer, E. W. (1967). Cortical activity preceding speech: Semantic specificity. *Nature, 216(5122)*, 1338-1339.

Schlesinger, B. (1962). Higher cerebral functions and their clinical disorders. New York: Grune and Stratton.

Schmidt, J. B. (1871). Casuistik, Gehörs- und Sprachstörung in Folge von Apoplexie. *Allg. Zschr. Psychiat., 27*, 304-306.

Schneider, A. M. (1966). Retention under spreading depression: A generalization decrement phenomenon. *J. Comp. Physiol. Psychol., 62(2)*, 317-319.

Schneider, A. M. (1967). Control of memory by spreading cortical depression: A case for stimulus control. *Psychol. Rev. 74(3)*, 201-215.

Schneider, A. M. (1968). Stimulus control and spreading cortical depression: Some problems reconsidered. *Psychol. Rev., 75(4)*, 353-358.

Schneider, A. M. and Behar, M. A. (1964). A chronic preparation for spreading cortical depression. *J. Exp. Anal. Behav., 7*, 350.

Schrier, A. and Sperry, R. W. (1959). Visuo-motor integration in split-brain cats. *Science, 129*, 1275-1276.

Semmes, J., Weinstein, S., Ghent, L. and Teuber, H. L. (1955). Spatial orientation in man after cerebral injury; analyses by locus of lesion. *J. Psychol., 39*, 227-244.

Semmes, J., Weinstein, S., Ghent, L. and Teuber, H. L. (1960). *Somatosensory changes after penetrating brain wounds in man.* Cambridge: Harvard University Press.

Semmes, J. and Mishkin, M. (1964). A search for cortical substrate of tactual memories. In *Functions of the corpus callosum,* ed. Ettlinger, E. G. London: Churchill.

Sergeev, B. F. (1964). Associative temporary connections in lower vertebrates. Proc. of the Xth Congress of All-Union Physiological Society, named after I. P. Pavlov. *Publ. Science, Moscow/Leningrad.* v. 2, p. 2, 263-264.

Serkov, F. N. and Makul'kin, R. F. (1965). Electrical activity of the brain after hemispherectomy. *Fed. Proc. Fed. Amer. Socs. Exp. Biol. (Transl. Suppl.), 24*, 443-449.

Shankweiler, D. (1966). Effects of temporal lobe damage on perception of dichotically presented melodies. *J. Comp. Physiol. Psychol., 62(1)*, 115-119.

Shankweiler, D. and Studdert-Kennedy, M. (1967). Identification of consonants and vowels presented to left and right ears. *Quart. J. Exp. Psychol., 19*, 59-63.

Shankweiler, D., Harris, K. S. and Taylor, M. L. (1968). Electromyographic studies of articulation in aphasia. *Arch. Phys. Med., 49*, 1-8.

Shannon, C. E. and Weaver, W. (1949). *The mathematical theory of communication.* Urbana IK: University of Illinois Press.

Shurrager, P. S. (1941). Specific functional relations ascribed to the agranular motor cortices, corpus callosum and contralateral and ipsilateral pyramidal tracts in conditioning and extinction. *Psychol. Bull., 38*, 570-571.

Siger, L. (1968). Gestures, the language of signs and human communication. *Amer. Ann. Deaf, 113*, 11-28.

Simon, J. R. (1964). Steadiness, handedness and hand preference. *Percept. Mot. Skills, 18*, 203-206.

Simon, J. R. (1967). Ear preference in a simple R.T. task. *J. Exp. Psychol., 75*, 49-55.

Sinclair, C. (1968). Ear dominance in preschool children. *Percept. Mot. Skills, 26*, 510.

Singer, W. (1969). Bilateral E.E.G. synchronization and interhemispheric transfer of somato-sensory and visual evoked potentials in chronic and acute split-brain preparations in the cat. *Electroenceph. Clin. Neurophysiol., 26*, 434.

Slager, V. T., Kelly, A. B. and Wagner, J. A. (1957). Congenital absence of the corpus callosum. *New Eng. J. Med., 256*, 1171-1176.

Sloan, N. and Jasper, H. H. (1950). The identity of spreading depression and 'suppression'. *Electroenceph. Clin. Neurophysiol., 2*, 59-78.

Smith, A. (1966). Intellectual functions in patients with lateralized frontal tumours. *J. Neurol. Neurosurg. Psychiat., 29(1),* 52-59.

Smith, A. (1966). Speech and other functions after left (dominant) hemispherectomy. *J. Neurol. Neurosurg. Psychiat., 29,* 467.

Smith, A. and Burklund, C. W. (1966). Dominant hemispherectomy: Preliminary report on neuropsychological sequelae. *Science, 153(3741),* 1280-1282.

Smith, A. and Burklund, C. W. (1967). Nondominant hemispherectomy: Neuropsychological implications for human brain functions. *Proc. of the 75th Annual Convention of the APA 1967, 2,* 103-104.

Smith, A. (1969). Nondominant hemispherectomy. *Neurology (Minneap.), 19,* 442-445.

Smith, K. U. (1947). Bilateral integrative action of the cerebral cortex in man in verbal association and sensori-motor coordination. *J. Exp. Psychol., 37,* 367-376.

Smith, K. U. (1951). Learning and the association pathways of the human cerebral cortex. *Science, 114,* 117-121.

Smith, K. U. and Akelaitis, A. J. (1942). Studies on the corpus callosum. I. Laterality in behaviour and bilateral motor organization in man before and after section of the corpus callosum. *Arch. Neurol. Psychiat. Chic., 47,* 519-543.

Sokolov, E. N. (1960). Neuronal models and the orienting reflex. In *The central nervous system and behaviour,* ed. Brazier, M. A. B. New York: Josiah Macy, Jr. Foundation.

Solursh, L. P., Margulies, A. I., Ashem, B. and Stasiak, E. A. (1965). The relationship of agenesis of the corpus callosum to perception and learning. *J. Nerv. Ment. Dis., 141,* 180-189.

Sparks, R. and Geschwind, N. (1968). Dichotic listening in man after section of neocortical commissures. *Cortex, 4(1),* 3-16.

Sperry, R. W. (1956). Experiments on perceptual integration in animals. *Psychiat. Res. Rep., 6,* 151-160.

Sperry, R. W. (1958). Corpus callosum and interhemispheric transfer in the monkey *(Macaca mulatta). Anat. Rec., 131,* 297.

Sperry, R. W. (1966). Brain bisection and mechanisms of consciousness. In *Brain and conscious experience,* ed. Eccles, J. C. New York: Springer Verlag.

Sperry, R. W. (1968a). Hemisphere deconnection and unity in conscious awareness. *Amer. Psychol., 23,* 723-733.

Sperry, R. W. (1968b). Mental unity following surgical disconnection of the cerebral hemispheres. *Harvey Lecture (1966-1967), 62,* 293-323.

Sperry, R. W. and Gazzaniga, M. S. (1966). Language following surgical disconnection of the hemispheres. In *Brain mechanisms underlying speech and language,* ed. Millikan, C. H. New York: Grune and Stratton.

Sperry, R. W. and Gazzaniga, M. S. (1967). Language following surgical disconnection of the hemispheres. In *Brain mechanisms underlying speech and language,* ed. Darley, F. L. New York: Grune and Stratton.

Sperry, R. W. and Green, S. M. (1964). Corpus callosum and perceptual integration of visual half fields. *Anat. Record, 148,* 339.

Squire, L. R. (1966). Transfer of habituation under spreading depression. *Psychonomic Science, 5(7),* 261-262.

Stark, R. (1961). An investigation of unilateral cerebral pathology with equated verbal and visual-spatial tasks. *J. Abnorm. Soc. Psychol., 62,* 282-287.

Stamm, J. S. and Sperry, R. W. (1957). Functions of corpus callosum in contralateral transfer of somesthetic discrimination in cats. *J. Comp. Physiol. Psychol., 50,* 138.

Stöer, W. F. H. (1940). Das optische System beim Wassermolch *(Triturus taeniatus). Acta Morph. Neerl. Scand., 3,* 178-195.

Straw, R. N. and Mitchell, C. L. (1967). Effect of section of the corpus callosum on cortical after-discharge patterns in the cat. *Proc. Soc. Exp. Biol. Med., 125,* 128-132.

Studdert-Kennedy, M., Liberman, A. M., Harris, K. S. and Cooper, F. S. (1970). Motor theory of speech perception: A reply to Lane's critical review. *Psych. Rev.,* Vol. 77, No. 3, 234-249.

Sugar, O. (1952). Congenital aphasia: an antomical and physiological approach. *J. Speech Hear. Dis., 17,* 301-304.

Sutton, L. R., Cohen, B. S. and Krusen, U. L. (1967). Nerve conduction studies in hemiplegia. *Arch. Phys. Med., 48,* 64-67.

Sutton, P. R. (1963). Handedness and facial asymmetry: lateral position of the nose in two racial groups. *Nature, 198,* 909.

Suzuki, H. and Uneoka, K. (1966). Effect of cortical spreading depression on operant behaviour in the rabbit. *Physiology and Behaviour, 1(4),* 301-304.

Swets, J. A. (ed.) (1964). *Signal detection and recognition by human observers.* New York: Wiley.

Tanner, W. P. and Swets, J. A. (1954). A decision-making theory of visual detection. *Psychol. Rev., 61,* 401-409.

Taylor, M. L. (1965). A measurement of functional communication in aphasia. *Arch. Phys. Med. Rehabil., 46(1-A),* 101-107.

Tapp, J. T. (1962). Reversible cortical depression and avoidance behaviour in the rat. *J. Comp. Physiol. Psychol., 55(3),* 306-308.

Terrace, H. S. (1959). The effects of retinal locus and attention on the perception of words. *J. Exp. Psychol., 58,* 382-385.

Teuber, H. L. (1962). Effects of brain wounds implicating right or left hemisphere in man. In *Interhemispheric relations and cerebral dominance.* ed. Mountcastle, V. B. Baltimore: Johns Hopkins Press.

Teuber, H. L., Battersby, W. and Bender, H. B. (1960). *Visual field defects after penetrating missile wounds of the brain.* Cambridge: Harvard University Press.

Teuber, H. L. and Diamond, S. (1956). Effects of brain injury in man on binaural localization of sounds. Paper read at 27th Annual Meeting of the Eastern Psychological Association, Atlantic City.

Teuber, H. L. and Weinstein, S. (1954). Performance on a formboard task after penetrating brain injury. *J. Psychol., 38,* 177-190.

Thompson, R. W. and Hjelle, L. A. (1965). Effects of stimulus and response complexity on learning under bilateral spreading depression. *J. Comp. Physiol. Psychol., 59,* 122-124.

Tilney, F. (1938). The hippocampus and its relation to the corpus callosum. *Bull. Neurol. Inst. N.Y., 7,* 1-77.

Travis, A. M. and Woolsey, C. (1956). Motor performance of monkeys. *Amer. J. Phys. Med., 35,* 273-310.

Travis, L. E. (1931). *Speech pathology.* New York: Appleton.

Travis, R. P. (1964). The role of spreading cortical depression in relating the amount of avoidance training in interhemispheric transfer. *J. Comp. Physiol. Psychol., 57,* 42-46.

Travis, R., Jr. and Sparks, D. (1963). The influence of unilateral and bilateral spreading depression during learning and subsequent relearning. *J. Comp. Physiol. Psychol., 56,* 56-59.

Treisman, A. M. (1960). Contextual cues in selective listening. *Quart. J. Exp. Psychol., 12,* 242-248.

Treisman, A. M. (1964). The effect of irrelevant material on the efficiency of selective listening. *Amer. J. Psychol.*, 77, 533-646.

Treisman, A. M. (1965). The effects of redundancy and familiarity on translating and repeating back a foreign and a native language. *Brit. J. Psychol.*, 56, 369-379.

Treisman, A. M. and Geffen, G. (1967). Selective attention: Perception or response. *Quart. J. Exp. Psychol.*, 19, 1-17.

Treisman, A. M. and Riley, G. (1969). Is selective attention selective perception or selective response. A further test. *J. Exp. Psychol.*, 79(1), 27-34.

Trescher, J. H. and Ford, F. R. (1937). Colloid cyst of third ventricle: report of a case: operative removal with section of posterior half of corpus callosum. *Arch. Neurol. Psychiat.*, 37, 959-973.

Trevarthen, C. (1962a). Exploring the neural mechanisms of mind. *Engn. Sci.*, 26, 15-24.

Trevarthen, C. (1962b). Double visual learning in split-brain monkeys. *Science*, 136, 258-259.

Trevarthen, C. (1963). Processus visuels intérhémisphériques localisés dans le tronc cérébral. *Compt. Rend. Soc. Biol.*, 157, 2019-2022.

Trevarthen, C. (1964). Functional interactions between the cerebral hemispheres of the split-brain monkey. In *Functions of the corpus callosum*, ed. Ettlinger, G. London: Churchill.

Tsai, L. and Maurer, S. (1930). Right handedness in white rats. *Science*, 72, 436-438.

Tschirgi, R. (1958). Spatial perception and central nervous system symmetry. *Arq. Neuro-psiquiat.*, 16, 364-366.

Tunturi, A. R. (1946). A study of the pathway from the medial geniculate body to the acoustic cortex in the dog. *Am. J. Physiol.*, 147, 311-319.

Turkewitz, G., Gordon, E. W. and Birch, H. G. (1965). Head turning in the human neonate: effect of prandial condition and lateral preference. *J. Comp. Physiol. Psychol.*, 59, 189-192.

Ueki, K. (1966). *Hemispherectomy in the human with special reference to the preservation of function.* Progress in Brain Research. 21B Correlative neurosciences. Part B: Clinical Studies, eds. Tokizane, T. and Schadé, J. P. pp. 285-338. Amsterdam: Elsevier.

Vaughan, H. G., Jr. and Katzman, R. (1964). Evoked response in visual disorders. *Annals N.Y. acad. Sci.*, 112(1), 305-319.

Vince, M. A. (1948). The intermittency of control movements and the psychological refractory period. *Brit. J. Psychol.*, 38, 149-157.

Vince, M. A. (1950). Some exceptions to the psychological refractory period in unskilled manual responses. M.R.C. Applied Psychology Research Unit Rep. No. 124/50.

Wada, J. (1949). A new method for the determination of the side of cerebral speech dominance. A preliminary report on the intracarotid injection of sodium amytal in man. *Med. Biol.*, 14, 221.

Wada, J. and Rasmussen, T. (1960). Intracarotid injection of sodium amytal for the lateralization of cerebral speech dominance. *J. Neurosurg.*, 17, 266-282.

Wagenen, W. P. von and Herren, R. Y. (1940). Surgical division of commissural pathways in the corpus callosum. *Arch. Neurol. Psychiat.*, 44, 740-759.

Walls, G. L. (1963). *The vertebrate eye and its adaptive radiation.* New York: Hafner.

Wapner, S. and Cirillo, L. (1968). Imitation of a model's hand movements: Age changes in transposition of left-right relations. *Child Dev.*, 39(3), 887-894.

Warren, J. M. (1953). Handedness in the rhesus monkey. *Science, 118,* 622-623.
Warren, J. M. (1958). The development of paw preferences in cats and monkeys. *J. Genet. Psychol., 93,* 229-236.
Warrington, E. K. and James, M. (1967). An experimental investigation of facial recognition in patients with unilateral cerebral lesions. *Cortex, 3(3),* 317-326.
Washburn, R. W. (1929). A study of the smiling and laughing of infants in the first year of life. *Genet. Psychol. Monogr., 6,* 396-537.
Webster, R. G. and Haslerud, G. M. (1964). Influence on extreme peripheral vision of attention to a visual or auditory task. *J. Exp. Psychol., 68,* 269-272.
Weinstein, E. A. (1964). Affections of speech with lesions of the non-dominant hemisphere. *Res. Publ. Ass. Res. Nerv. Ment. Dis., 42,* 220-225.
Weinstein, E. A. and Kahn, R. L. (1955). *Denial of illness: symbolic and physiological aspects.* Springfield, Illnois: C. Thomas.
Weinstein, E. A. and Keller, N. J. A. (1963). Linguistic patterns of misnaming in brain injury. *J. Neuropsychol., 1,* 79-90.
Weinstein, S. (1955a). Tactile size judgement after penetrating injury to the brain. *J. Comp. Physiol. Psychol., 48,* 106-109.
Weinstein, S. (1955b). Time error in weight judgement after brain injury. *J. Comp. Physiol. Psychol., 48,* 203-207.
Weinstein, S. (1962). Intellectual and perceptual functions in man. In *Interhemispheric relations and cerebral dominance,* ed. Mountcastle, V. B. Baltimore: Johns Hopkins Press.
Weinstein, S. (1963). Tactile sensitivity of the phalanges. *Percept. Mot. Skills, 14,* 351-354.
Weinstein, S. (1964). Deficits concomitant with aphasia or lesions of either cerebral hemisphere. *Cortex, 1(2),* 154-167.
Weinstein, S. and Sersen, E. A. (1961). Tactual sensitivity as a function of handedness and laterality. *J. Comp. Physiol. Psychol., 54,* 665-669.
Weiss, S., Levy, I., Smith, D. and O'Leary, J. L. (1956). Loss of right hemisphere due to natural causes. *Electroenceph. Clin. Neurophysiol., 8,* 682-684.
Welford, A. T. (1952). The "psychological refractory period" and the timing of high-speed performance. *Brit. J. Psychol., 43,* 2-19.
Welford, A. T. (1958). *Ageing and human skill.* Oxford University Press for the Nuffield Foundation.
Welford, A. T. (1967). Single channel operation in the brain. *Acta Psychol., 27,* 5-22.
Welford, A. T. (1968). *Fundamentals of skill.* London: Methuen.
Welker, W. I. and Seidenstein, S. (1959). Somatic sensory representation in the cerebral cortex of the racoon *(Procyon lotor). J. Comp. Neurol., 111,* 469-501.
Wernicke, C. (1874). *Der aphasische Symptomencomplex. Eine psychologische Studie auf anatomischer Basis.* Breslau: Cohn and Weigert.
Wernicke, C. (1906). *Grundriss der Psychiatrie in klinischen Vorlesungen.* 2nd rev. edition. Leipzig: Thieme.
Whatmore, G. B. and Kleitman, N. (1946). The role of sensory and motor cortex in escape and avoidance conditioning in dogs. *Amer. J. Physiol., 146,* 282-292.
White, M. J. (1970). Signal detection analysis of laterality differences: some preliminary data, free of recall and report sequence characteristics. *J. Exp. Psychol., 83(1),* 174-176.
Whitteridge, D. (1965). Area 18 and the vertical meridian of the visual field. In *Functions of the corpus callosum,* ed. Ettlinger, G. London: J. & A. Churchill.
Wiener, N. (1948). *Cybernetics.* New York: Wiley.
Wigan, A. L. (1844). *The duality of the mind: A new view of insanity.* London: Longman, Brown, Green and Longman.

Winocur, G. (1965). Bilateral spreading depression and avoidance learning in rats. *Psychonomic Science, 3(3),* 107-108.

Wolff, B. B. and Jarvik, M. E. (1964). Relationship between superficial and deep somatic thresholds of pain with a note on handedness. *Amer. J. Psychol., 77,* 589-599.

Wyke, M. (1966). Postural am drift associated with brain lesions in man. *Arch. Neurol. Chicago, 15,* 329-334.

Wyke, M. (1967). Effect of brain lesions on the rapidity of arm movement. *Neurology, 17,* 1113-1120.

Yates, A. J. (1965). Delayed auditory feedback and shadowing. *Quart. J. Exp. Psychol., 17,* 125-131.

Young, J. Z. (1962). Why do we have two brains? In *Interhemispheric relations and cerebral dominance,* ed. Mountcastle, V. B. Baltimore: Johns Hopkins Press.

Zangwill, O. L. (1960). *Cerebral dominance and its relation to psychological function.* Edinburgh: Oliver and Boyd.

Zangwill, O. L. (1963). Cerebral localization of psychological function. *The Advancement of Science, 20, 86,* 335; *87,* 466.

Zangwill, O. L. (1964). The brain and disorders of communication. The current status of cerebral dominance. *Res. Publ. Ass. Nerv. Ment. Dis., 42,* 103-118.

Zangwill, O. L. (1967). Speech and the minor hemisphere. *Acta Neurol. Psychiat. Belg., 67(11),* 1013-1020.

Zavarzin, A. A. (1941). *Ocherki po evoliutsionnoi gistologii nervnoi sistemy.* Moscow/Leningrad: Medgiz.

Zollinger, R. (1935). Removal of left cerebral hemisphere: report of a case. *Arch. Neurol. Psychiat., 34,* 1055-1064.

Index